KETTLEBELL EXERCISE ENCYCLOPEDIA

Kettlebell exercises and variations in one handy book with detailed photos.

VOLUME 3/5: Press, Push-up, Row, and Snatch

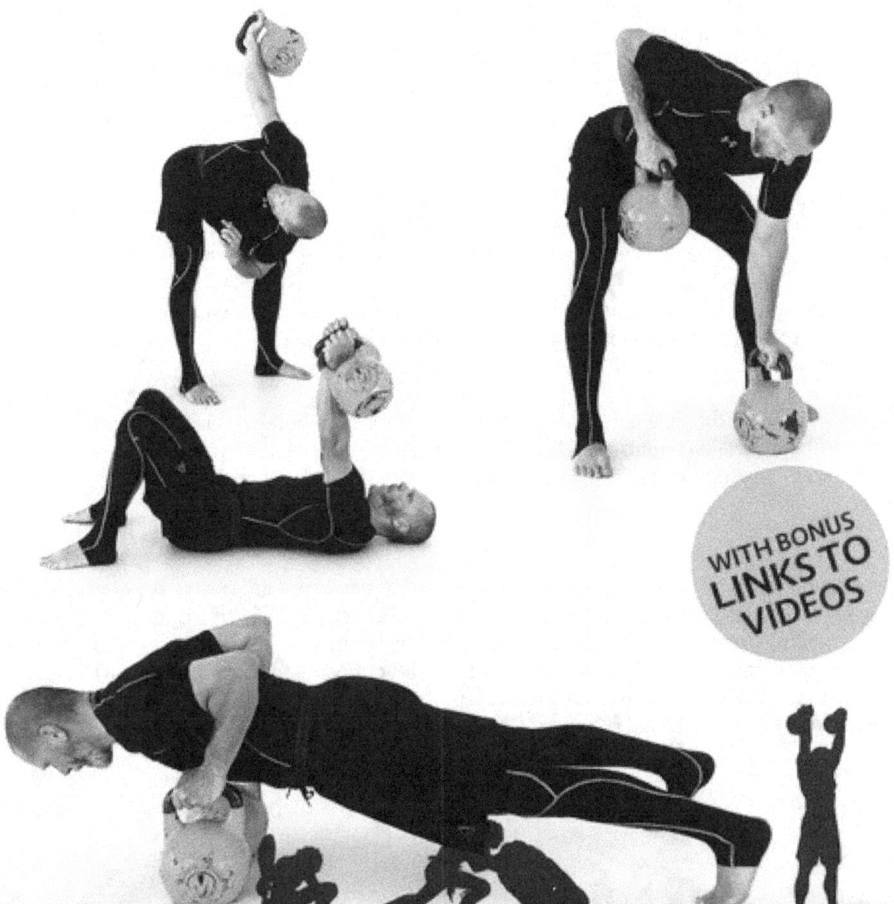

WITH BONUS LINKS TO VIDEOS

By Taco Fleur from Cavemantraining

Kettlebell Exercise Encyclopedia

Kettlebell training is a form of resistance training with the kettlebell. This book covers all kettlebell exercises with photos, descriptions, and some having step-by-step instructions. The information in this book will allow you to pick exercises and create your own kettlebell workout and/or verify that you're doing the exercises you're already doing, correctly.

The encyclopedia covers kettlebells cleans, swings, presses, lifts, snatches, squats, lunges, rows, getups, windmills, isometric exercises, isolation exercises, multi-planar exercises, combos, and more. Each subject has just enough information to keep it basic and understandable.

There are several volumes of the encyclopedia with each volume covering a set of kettlebell exercise categories. The encyclopedia is updated every 3 to 6 months with newly added exercises. If you purchased all volumes then you're entitled to download an updated digital copy from *Cavemantraining.com*, please visit go.cavemantraining.com/kbe-updates for details.

The layout and indexing of this book explained. Some exercises will have more information than others as they'll be the base for other variations. To give an example, the swing high pull contains a swing and a pull, but the swing is not explained as this would be duplicating the swing previously explained, plus, one can use different variations of the swing with the pull added.

The introduction and additional information will be repeated for each volume as it applies to all exercises and some readers might only want to purchase one particular volume that covers their subject of interest.

Compiling a resource that has each and every variation of kettlebell exercises in existence is a task that's daunting and takes time, therefore, some exercise names are listed but won't have any content, they are awaiting to be completed in the next update of the encyclopedia.

If an exercise is done with two kettlebells, and you only have two uneven kettlebells with not too much weight difference between them, let's say up to 8kg/17.6lbs max, use them. There is absolutely nothing wrong with using uneven weights, more difficult in most cases, yes, but bad, no. It does not create muscle imbalance either, in fact, the opposite, assuming you don't do anything unsound like training for months with the lighter weight on your left, and the heavier on the right side. Swap weights after a round or two.

About the Author

My name is Taco Fleur, and I'm a Russian Girevoy Sport Institute Kettlebell Coach, IKFF Certified Kettlebell Trainer, Kettlebell Level 1 + 2 Trainer, Kettlebell Science and Application, CrossFit Level 1 Trainer, CrossFit Judges Certificate, CrossFit Programming Certificate, MMA Conditioning Level 1, MMA Fitness Level 1 + 2, Punchfit Trainer and Plyometrics Trainer Certified, with a purple belt in Brazilian Jiu-Jitsu. Author on BoxRox and featured in 4 issues of the Iron Man magazine. I have owned and set-up 3 functional kettlebell gyms in Australia and Vietnam, and lived in the Netherlands, Australia, Vietnam, and Thailand. I'm currently living in Spain.

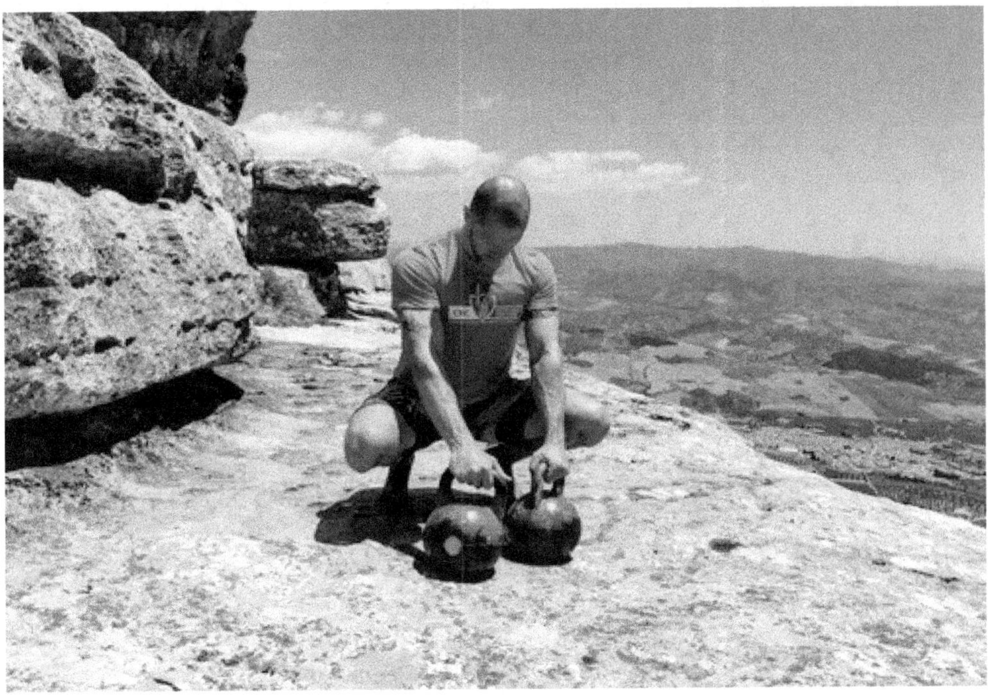

The first thing I'd like you to know about me is that I do **not** know everything, I don't pretend to know everything, and I never will. I'm on a path of life-long learning. I believe there is always something to learn from someone, no matter who they are. I've been physically active since the day I arrived on this earth in 1973. I got serious about training in 1999, touched a kettlebell for the first time in 2004, and got serious about kettlebell training in 2009. I'm here to do what I love most, and that is to share my knowledge with the world.

Some of my personal bests are 1 hour unbroken clean and jerk with a 16kg; 45 minutes unbroken clean and jerk with a 20kg; 400 burpees performed within one hour; 500 kettlebell snatches, 500 swings, and 500 double-unders completed in one session; 250 alternating dead clean and presses in one session with 20kg; 200 pull-ups in one session; 200 unbroken kettlebell swings with a 28kg; most kettlebell swings completed in one session with a 28kg (1,501); most total kettlebell swings done in 28 days with a 28kg (11,111); windmill with a 40kg kettlebell; lugged a kettlebell up a 3,479m mountain; 160kg dead lift; 100 snatches on sand with a 24kg kettlebell; 85kg Olympic Squat Snatch; 300 unbroken clean and jerk with 20kg kettlebell; 10 minute unbroken clean and jerk 80 reps with 2 x 16kg kettlebells; 532 unbroken snatches and achieved rank 2 in kettlebell sport. I mention these PBs not to boast but to demonstrate that I have a good understanding of technique and movement across different areas.

My own training and goals are geared around GPP (General Physical Preparedness) which involves kettlebell training, calisthenics, and CrossFit. I like high-volume reps but also like greasing the groove now and again. My main goals are to remains as agile as possible, remaining mobile, training in as many planes of movements as possible, and learning as many different exercise combinations and movements as possible while having fun and enjoying Brazilian Jiu-Jitsu. I'm no Arnold Schwarzenegger and never will be, but strength is not solely defined by physical appearance and huge bulging muscles.

You can read more about my training, philosophy, and other ramblings on the Cavemantraining website, www.cavemantraining.com, and on the Cavemantraining YouTube channel, bit.ly/youtube-cavemantraining, which as of this writing has over 37,000 subscribers and more than 5 million views.

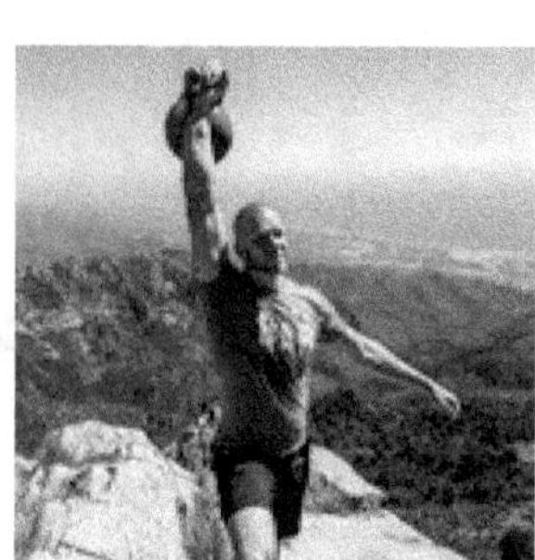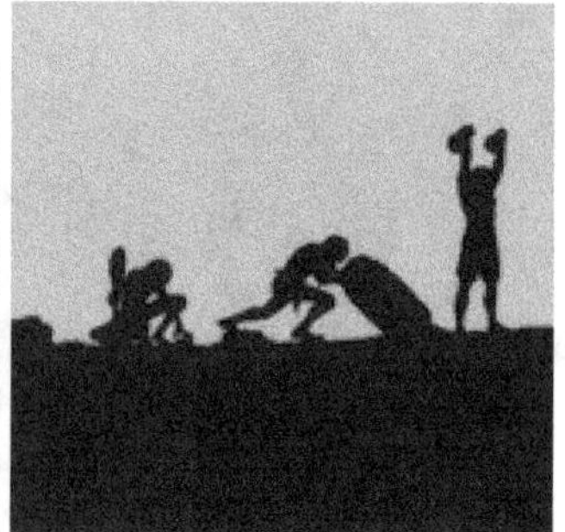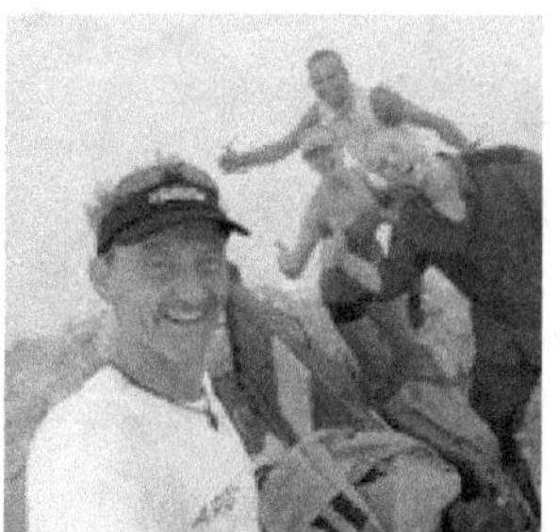

Add me: Facebook.com/taco.fleur or Facebook.com/coach.taco.fleur
Instagram: *@realcavemantraining*
Reddit: *u/cavemankettlebells*

Facebook.com/Cavemantraining or Facebook.com/Cavemantraining.Magazine
for up-to-date articles and news.

Please note that this material may not be reproduced or publicized elsewhere without the written consent of the author me@tacofleur.com.

If you bought this as a PDF/electronic copy, it is digitally signed and password protected with identifiable information.

All Cavemantraining owned images are copyrighted © Cavemantraining™

Note: Most of the <u>kettlebell stock images</u> used in this book have literally been created with blood, sweat, and tears - I'm talking about lugging kettlebells for hours up mountains, through canyons, running out of water to drink, etc. Please respect the effort that has gone into producing the photos.

Photos are available for purchase, or in some cases made available for educational purposes with appropriate credits/links in return.

CAVEMANTRAINING

Table of Contents

Kettlebell Novice

If you came to this book as a kettlebell novice I can highly recommend you first check out the information on kettlebell grips and kettlebell anatomy toward the end of the book.

Links

Please note that any links in this book are case-sensitive, this means that if you would type in go.cavemantraining.com/*KBE-VID-001* instead of go.cavemantraining.com/*kbe-vid-001* then the link will provide an error message.

Definitions

- **Athlete**
  A person who is proficient in sports and other forms of physical exercise

- **ROM**
  Range of motion—the full and safe movement potential of a joint

- **Joint**
  A structure in the human body at which two parts of the skeleton are fitted together

- **Flexion**
  The action of bending of a limb or joint

- **Extension**
  The action of moving a limb from a bent to a straight position

- **Mobility**
  The ability to move or be moved freely and easily

- **Flexibility**
  The quality of bending easily without breaking

- **Anterior**
  Located at the front of the body

- **Posterior**
  Located at the back of the body

- **Lateral**
  Toward one side or other of the body

- **1RM**
  One repetition maximum—the maximum weight you can lift for one repetition

- **Humerus**
  The bone of the upper arm or forelimb, forming joints at the shoulder and the elbow

- **Scapulae**
  Plural for scapula (shoulder blade)

- **Spine**
  24 discs

- **Cervical**
  7 discs in the spine ranging from 1 to 7

- **Thoracic**
  12 discs in the spine ranging from 8 to 19

- **Lumbar**
  5 discs in the spine ranging from 20 to 24

- ***MMC***
  Mind muscle connection

Ankle dorsiflexion is where the toes are brought closer to the shin. This decreases the angle between the dorsum of the foot and the leg. For example, when walking on the heels the ankle is described as being in dorsiflexion.

Ankle plantar flexion is the opposite of dorsiflexion. Plantar flexion is the movement which decreases the angle between the sole of the foot and the back of the leg. For example, the movement when depressing a car pedal or standing on the tiptoes can be described as plantar flexion.

Pronation at the forearm is a rotational movement where the hand and upper arm are turned inwards. Pronation of the foot refers to turning of the sole outwards so that weight is borne on the medial part of the foot.

Supination of the forearm occurs when the forearm or palm are rotated outwards. Supination of the foot refers to turning of the sole of the foot inwards, shifting weight to the lateral edge.

Flexion and *extension* are examples of angular motions, in which two axes of a joint are brought closer together or moved further apart. For example, elbow flexion (flex the biceps) is where you bring your hand closer toward your shoulder, and the opposite, elbow extension is where you arm moves toward being straight.

Torque, moment, or moment of force is rotational force. Just as a linear force is a push or a pull, a torque can be thought of as a twist to an object. In three dimensions, the torque is a pseudo-vector; for point particles, it is given by the cross product of the position vector (distance vector) and the force vector. Needless to say, torque is complex. There is always some form of torque happening during training, for the purpose of this book, I use the word to define more rotational pull being present than in other exercises, i.e. the exercise requires the body to resist more against a pulling force that wants to twist the body.

Dead refers to the object not moving, not having any momentum at all before being lifted, or cleaned in our case. Dead is not to be confused with Deadlifting, which means lifting a dead weight from the ground to hanging in standing position, this can be done with a hip hinge or with a squatting movement.

Exercise Category

When looking at kettlebell exercises they can be categorized into a parent exercise—the base exercise—and its variations, following are the most common exercises to categorize the variations by.

- Kettlebell Carry
- Kettlebell Clean
- Kettlebell Curl
- Kettlebell Getup
- Kettlebell Isometrics
- Kettlebell Kneeling
- Kettlebell Lift
- Kettlebell Lunge
- Kettlebell Press
- Kettlebell Push-up
- Kettlebell Step-up
- Kettlebell Row
- Kettlebell Snatch
- Kettlebell Squat
- Kettlebell Swing

Kettlebell Carry

Support and move a kettlebell from one place to another. The support can be provided in the form of overhead, racked, hanging, or a mixture of aforementioned methods.

Kettlebell Clean

A kettlebell clean is an explosive lower-body powered movement that lifts a kettlebell from a lower position to a higher position which is called racking position. The clean can be performed from the ground (dead), hanging position, or a during a ballistic movement like the swing.

Anytime a clean is performed with a swing, then that swing can be either one of the following movements, hip hinge swing, pendulum swing, or squat swing.

Kettlebell Curl

Curl refers to the curling motion which in exercise can be performed with the elbow or knee joint, i.e. Biceps Curls or Leg Curls. Think flexion and extension of the elbow joint, or decreasing and increasing the angle of the elbow joint. When it comes to kettlebell training the common curling exercise used is the biceps curl, although technically speaking the leg curl could be performed laying down and the foot through the window of the kettlebell.

Kettlebell Get-up

To get up into a fully erect position any way possible from laying flat on the floor. This can be done with 1 or 2 kettlebells positioned overhead or racked.

Kettlebell Isometrics

Isometric relates to muscular action in which tension is developed without contraction of the muscle. There is no movement, action, or change, also known as static. A good example of an isometric exercise is the plank or iron cross. Isometrics can also be mixed with dynamic exercise, for example, a squat with frontal hold.

Kettlebell Kneeling

To kneel means to be in or assume a position in which the body is supported by a knee or the knees. You can perform movements into kneeling positions like surrenders or you can perform exercises in which you remain in kneeling position like kneeling hip thrusts.

Kettlebell Lift

To lift something means to raise to a higher position or level. In effect, almost all kettlebell exercises could be thought of like a lift, i.e. snatch, press, clean, swing, etc. However, we're going to classify a lift as a movement in which the kettlebell is brought from a low to a higher position via a slow movement. We're excluding explosive movements as they have their own classifications, i.e. press, snatch, clean, and swing.

Kettlebell Lunge

To define the lunge a few assumptions will be made. The dictionary defines the word as making a sudden forward thrust with part of the body, in our context that part of the body would be the leg. A lunge is also the basic attacking move in fencing, which is very similar to the lunge exercise as we know it. The lunge as we know it not only moves forward but all different directions, back (reverse), side, etc. The difference between the lunge used in fencing and exercise is that the back knee usually bends and gently taps the floor to set a standard for depth.

Kettlebell Press

The press and push movement are very similar when you look at the arms, they're always extending, whether overhead or above the chest (laying down), however, there is a clear difference between the two. With the press, you exert physical force on the kettlebell to move it away from you rather than to move yourself away from it (push).

Kettlebell Push-up

Similar to the press, you exert physical force on the kettlebell, but in this case, it's in order to move yourself away from it. A push-up done on the floor would be pushing yourself away from the floor. If you take the same push-up position and turn it around—laying flat—and perform the same movement it becomes as press as you're moving the object away from yourself.

Kettlebell Step-up

A step-up is performed by placing one foot onto a higher plateau and pushing yourself up by exerting force and extending the working leg. You can perform step-ups on box jumps, stairs, or other suitable objects.

Kettlebell Row

When looking at the movement in boat rowing it's always a pull and push off the oar. In the context of kettlebell training, a row is always a pull as gravity replaces the push. A row has to be performed in such a way that you're acting directly against gravity. The focus of the kettlebell row are the posterior muscles of the upper back.

Kettlebell Snatch

A snatch is a movement in which the kettlebell rapidly raised from a lower position—always below the hips—to above the head in one continuous smooth explosive movement. An example of a few common start positions are dead, hanging, and swinging.

Kettlebell Squat

The squat is a movement in which three joints flex, namely the ankle, knee, and hip joints. During the movement, the objective is to get the hips as low to the ground as possible while keeping the shoulders as high as possible. The squat can be performed in with the kettlebell(s) overhead, racked, or dead, however, when dead, it will be moved to the category of a lift.

Kettlebell Swing

A swing takes place when an object moves back and forth or from side to side while suspended. The swing is the foundation for many other exercises, such as the clean and snatch. The swing can be actioned as a pull or pendulum. The most common variation outside of the sport world is the pulling version whereas in the sport world it's the opposite and the pendulum is common.

List by Name

The following index is all kettlebell exercises by name. Note that not all variations are included in this book. The first column is the name, the second column is the variation, combine the two together and you have the full name, for example, *Carry Racked* would become *Racked Carry*. If it's single-arm and single kettlebell then it can be the left or right side and one arm is not working. If it's double-hand and single kettlebell then both hands are holding on to the kettlebell. If it's double-hand and double kettlebell then both sides have a kettlebell. If the hand is marked as alternating then that's a variation where the kettlebell goes from one side to the other.

Name Variation	Hand	Kettlebell
Carry Racked	Single	Single
Carry Racked	Double	Double
Carry Goblet	Double	Single
Carry Overhead	Single	Single
Carry Overhead	Double	Double
Carry Suitcase	Single	Single
Carry Suitcase	Double	Double
Carry Waiter	Single	Single
Carry Waiter	Double	Double
Clean Assisted Dead	Single	Single
Clean Assisted Hang	Single	Single
Clean Assisted Swing	Single	Single
Clean Assisted Dead Swing	Single	Single
Clean Dead	Single	Single
Clean Dead	Alternating	Single
Clean Dead	Double	Double
Clean Hang	Single	Single
Clean Hang	Alternating	Single
Clean Hang	Double	Double
Clean Gorilla	Double	Double
Clean Swing	Single	Single
Clean Swing	Alternating	Single
Clean Swing	Double	Single
Clean Swing	Double	Double
Clean Pendulum	Single	Single
Clean Pendulum	Alternating	Single

Name	Variation	Hand	Kettlebell
Clean	Pendulum	Double	Double
Clean	Half Circular	Single	Single
Clean	Circular	Single	Single
Clean	Goblet	Double	Single
Clean	Horn	Double	Single
Clean	Bottoms-up Horn	Double	Single
Clean	Suitcase	Single	Single
Clean	Suitcase	Double	Double
Clean	Suitcase	Alternating	Double
Clean	Suitcase Hang	Single	Single
Clean	Suitcase Hang	Double	Double
Clean	Suitcase Hang	Alternating	Double
Clean	Lawnmower	Single	Single
Clean	Lawnmower	Double	Double
Clean	Lawnmower	Double	Single
Curl	Conventional	Single	Single
Curl	Conventional	Double	Single
Curl	Conventional	Double	Double
Curl	Conventional	Alternating	Double
Curl	Hammer	Single	Single
Curl	Hammer	Double	Single
Curl	Hammer	Double	Double
Curl	Squat Dead	Single	Single
Curl	Squat Dead	Double	Double
Curl	Gorilla	Single	Single
Curl	Gorilla	Alternating	Double
Curl	Gorilla	Double	Double
Curl	Bent Side	Single	Single
Getup	Turkish Lunge	Single	Single
Getup	Turkish Squat	Single	Single
Getup	Racked	Double	Double
Getup	Shin Box Racked	Single	Single
Getup	Shin Box Racked	Double	Double
Getup	Shin Box Overhead	Single	Single

Name	Variation	Hand	Kettlebell
Getup	Shin Box Overhead	Double	Double
Isometrics	Crucifix	Double	Double
Isometrics	Frontal Hold	Double	Single
Isometrics	L-sit	Double	Double
Isometrics	Spartan Side Plank	Single	Single
Lift	Racked Deadlift	Double	Double
Lift	Hang Squat/Hip Hinge	Single	Single
Lift	Hang Squat/Hip Hinge	Double	Single
Lift	Hang Squat/Hip Hinge	Double	Double
Lift	Dead Squat/Hip Hinge	Single	Single
Lift	Dead Squat/Hip Hinge	Alternating	Single
Lift	Dead Squat/Hip Hinge	Double	Single
Lift	Dead Squat/Hip Hinge	Double	Double
Lift	Suitcase	Single	Single
Lift	Suitcase	Alternating	Double
Lift	Suitcase	Double	Double
Lift	Sumo Dead Squat/Hip Hinge	Single	Single
Lift	Sumo Dead Squat/Hip Hinge	Double	Single
Lift	Sumo Dead Squat/Hip Hinge	Alternating	Single
Lift	Sumo Dead Squat/Hip Hinge	Double	Double
Lift	Dead Stiff-legged	Single	Single
Lift	Dead Stiff-legged	Double	Double
Lift	Dead Stiff-legged	Alternating	Double
Lunge	Forward/Reverse Racked	Single	Single
Lunge	Forward/Reverse Racked	Double	Single
Lunge	Forward/Reverse Racked	Double	Double
Lunge	Forward/Reverse Overhead	Single	Single
Lunge	Forward/Reverse Overhead	Double	Double
Lunge	Curtsy Racked	Single	Single
Lunge	Curtsy Racked	Double	Single
Lunge	Curtsy Racked	Double	Double
Lunge	Curtsy Overhead	Single	Single
Lunge	Curtsy Overhead	Double	Double
Press	Front/Hybrid/Side	Single	Single

Name	Variation	Hand	Kettlebell
Press	Front/Hybrid/Side	Alternating	Double
Press	Front/Hybrid/Side	Double	Double
Press	Rear	Single	Single
Press	Seesaw	Double	Double
Press	Bent Side	Single	Single
Press	Push	Single	Single
Press	Push	Double	Double
Press	Sots	Single	Single
Press	Sots	Alternating	Double
Press	Sots	Double	Double
Press	Seated	Single	Single
Press	Seated	Alternating	Double
Press	Seated	Double	Double
Press	Chest	Single	Single
Press	Chest	Alternating	Double
Press	Chest	Double	Double
Press	Spiral	Single	Single
Row	Bent-over Lunge (Diff. angles)	Single	Single
Row	Bent-over (Diff. angles)	Single	Single
Row	Bent-over (Diff. angles)	Alternating	Double
Row	Bent-over (Diff. angles)	Double	Double
Row	Renegade	Double	Double
Snatch	Half Hip Hinge/Squat/Pendulum	Single	Single
Snatch	Half Hip Hinge/Squat/Pendulum	Alternating	Single
Snatch	Half Hip Hinge/Squat/Pendulum	Double	Double
Snatch	Full Hip Hinge/Squat/Pendulum	Single	Single
Snatch	Full Hip Hinge/Squat/Pendulum	Alternating	Single
Snatch	Full Hip Hinge/Squat/Pendulum	Double	Double
Snatch	Dead Half	Single	Single
Snatch	Dead Half	Alternating	Single
Snatch	Dead Half	Double	Double
Snatch	Dead Full	Single	Single
Snatch	Dead Full	Alternating	Single
Snatch	Dead Full	Double	Double

Name	Variation	Hand	Kettlebell
Squat	Racked	Single	Single
Squat	Racked	Double	Single
Squat	Racked	Double	Double
Squat	Deck	Double	Single
Squat	Pistol	Double	Single
Squat	Goblet	Double	Single
Squat	Overhead	Single	Single
Squat	Overhead	Double	Double
Squat	Back	Single	Single
Squat	Back	Double	Double
Squat	Cossack Racked	Single	Single
Squat	Cossack Racked	Double	Double
Squat	Cossack Overhead	Single	Single
Squat	Cossack Overhead	Double	Double
Squat	Thruster	Single	Single
Squat	Thruster	Double	Double
Squat	Hindu Racked	Single	Single
Squat	Hindu Racked	Double	Double
Squat	Hindu Overhead	Single	Single
Squat	Hindu Overhead	Double	Double
Swing	Hip Hinge/Squat/Pendulum	Single	Single
Swing	Hip Hinge/Squat/Pendulum	Alternating	Single
Swing	Hip Hinge/Squat/Pendulum	Double	Double
Swing	American	Double	Single
Swing	Atlas	Single	Single
Swing	Atlas	Double	Single
Swing	Short Lever	Double	Single
Swing	Gorilla	Single	Single
Swing	Gorilla	Double	Single
Swing	Gorilla	Double	Double
Swing	Power	Double	Single
Jerk	Conventional	Single	Single
Jerk	Conventional	Double	Double
Jerk	Split	Single	Single

Name Variation	Hand	Kettlebell
Jerk Split	Double	Double
Jerk Squat	Single	Single
Jerk Squat	Double	Double

The objective was to keep the list brief as there are plenty more variations than those listed. Just by changing up the grip on a clean you have a variation, for example, a dead clean with a waiters grip would become a waiters clean, a swing clean with an open palm would become an open palm swing clean, and so on. I purposely chosen not to do that with the above list. There is a list online which has more variation if you're interested.

http://bit.ly/kettlebell-exercise-list

List With Goal

The following list are all kettlebell exercises listed with their goal. The goals are generalized as the most common goals used for those exercises, but not meaning that's all they're good for. It should also be noted that most goals can change through programming. With the goals being:

- Muscular strength
- Cardiovascular endurance
  - Aerobic
  - Anaerobic
- Flexibility
- Balance
- Stability
- Mobility
- Agility
- Power
- Speed
- Cardiovascular endurance
- Muscular endurance
- Core

Cardiovascular Endurance

Cardiovascular endurance is how efficiently your heart, blood vessels, and lungs supply oxygen-rich blood to working muscles during physical activity for a prolonged period of time, usually for more than 90 seconds. You improve your cardiovascular endurance when you improve the capacity of the muscles to extract oxygen from the bloodstream to produce energy. Your cardiovascular endurance is improved when you can maintain an increased heart rate and breathing rate for a longer period of time than you were previously capable.

Balance

Balance is your ability to maintain an even distribution of weight enabling you to remain upright and steady during movement or static position.

Stability

Although often confused, stability is not the same as balance. Stability is the ability to prevent something from moving, it requires strength and a good mind-muscle connection.

Agility

Agility is the ability to move quickly and easily.

Power

Power is a combination of speed and strength.

Speed

Speed is very similar to power with the biggest difference being that the weight used is much lighter so to be able to maintain high-speed contractions with low resistance.

Muscular Endurance

Muscular endurance is a particular muscle's ability to continuously contract against a given resistance. A good example of this is the iron cross exercise in which your whole body is engaged and contracted, the longer you're able to stay in this position the greater your muscular endurance is. In other words, it defines how fatigue-resistant particular muscles are.

Muscular Strength

Muscular strength is the ability to perform one repetition at your maximal intensity. In other words, the amount of force particular muscles can produce in one, all-out effort.

Flexibility

The ability of a muscle or muscle groups to lengthen passively through a range of motion.

Mobility

Mobility is a combination of qualities that make it easy to come in and out of maximum range of any given muscle. Some qualities but not limited to are stability, strength, mind-muscle connection, etc.

Core

The muscles that attach to the spine and pelvis are referred to as the core muscles. Just about any exercise done while standing places a demand on the core muscles, but there are those that place and increased demand and those will be categorized here.

Name	Variation	Goal
Carry	Racked/Goblet	Muscular endurance, muscular strength, core
Carry	Overhead	Muscular endurance, muscular strength, core, stability, flexibility
Carry	Suitcase	Muscular endurance, muscular strength, core, stability
Clean	Assisted	Technique, drilling
Clean	Dead/Hang	Muscular strength, cardiovascular endurance, flexibility, power, muscular endurance, core
Clean	Gorilla	Muscular strength, cardiovascular endurance (anaerobic), power, core
Clean	Swing	Muscular strength, cardiovascular endurance (aerobic/anaerobic), core
Clean	Pendulum	Cardiovascular endurance (aerobic), muscular endurance, core
Clean	Suitcase/Suitcase Hang	Muscular strength, cardiovascular endurance, flexibility, power, muscular endurance, core
Curl	Conventional/Hammer	Muscular strength
Curl	Squat Dead/Gorilla/Bent Side	Muscular strength, flexibility
Getup	Turkish Lunge/Turkish Squat/Racked/Shin Box Racked/Shin Box Overhead	Muscular strength, muscular endurance, flexibility, mobility, stability, core
Isometrics	Crucifix/Frontal Hold/L-sit/Spartan Side Plank	Muscular strength, muscular endurance, stability, core
Lift	All variations	Muscular strength, flexibility, core
Lunge	Forward Racked	Muscular strength, flexibility, stability, core, explosive strength
Lunge	Reverse Racked	Muscular strength, flexibility, stability, core
Lunge	Curtsy Racked/Curtsy Overhead	Muscular strength, muscular endurance, flexibility, mobility, stability, core
Press	Front/Hybrid/Side	Muscular strength, flexibility, core
Press	Rear	Muscular strength, flexibility, mobility, core
Press	Seesaw	Muscular strength, muscular

Name	Variation	Goal
		endurance, flexibility, mobility, core
Press	Bent Side	Muscular strength, flexibility, mobility, core
Press	Push	Muscular strength, cardiovascular endurance, flexibility, power, core
Press	Sots	Muscular strength, muscular endurance, flexibility, mobility, stability, core
Press	Seated	Muscular strength, muscular endurance, flexibility
Press	Chest	Muscular strength
Press	Spiral	Muscular strength, muscular endurance, flexibility, mobility, stability, core
Row	Bent-over Lunge (Diff. angles)	Muscular strength, muscular endurance, flexibility, stability
Row	Bent-over (Diff. angles)/Renegade	Muscular strength, muscular endurance, flexibility, stability, core
Snatch	Half Hip Hinge/Squat	Power, muscular strength, muscular endurance, flexibility, cardiovascular endurance (aerobic/anaerobic), core
Snatch	Half Pendulum	Muscular endurance, cardiovascular endurance (aerobic), core
Snatch	Dead Half/Dead Full	Explosive strength, power, flexibility, cardiovascular endurance (anaerobic), muscular strength, core
Squat	Racked/Goblet/Overhead/Back	Muscular strength, muscular endurance, flexibility, core
Squat	Deck	Mobility, flexibility
Squat	Pistol	Muscular strength, muscular endurance, flexibility, core, stability, balance
Squat	Thruster	Muscular strength, power, muscular endurance, cardiovascular endurance (anaerobic), flexibility
Squat	Cossack Overhead/Cossack Racked/ Hindu Racked/Hindu Overhead	Muscular strength, muscular endurance, flexibility, stability, mobility, core
Swing	Hip Hinge/Squat/Power	Muscular strength, power, cardiovascular endurance (aerobic/anaerobic), flexibility, core

Name	Variation	Goal
Swing	Pendulum	Cardiovascular endurance (aerobic), core
Swing	American	Muscular strength, cardiovascular endurance (aerobic/anaerobic), flexibility, core
Swing	Atlas/Gorilla	Muscular strength, cardiovascular endurance, flexibility, core
Jerk	Conventional/Split/Squat	Muscular strength, cardiovascular endurance (aerobic/anaerobic), flexibility, core

Common Kettlebell References

Following are common kettlebell references used within many other exercises and thus important to list upfront so that it's easy to understand when referenced to later.

Hyperextension

What is Hip (Hyper)extension?

Our definition for hyperextension is most likely different from other writings you might have encountered. Haven written over 10 books and courses it has become obvious that the following definition of hyperextension works better for clarity and avoiding addition descriptions. Caveat: The hyperextension definition that follows should only be considered under the context of Cavemantraining material.

Hip flexion is where you pull the top of the pelvis down towards the ground, and extension is the opposite. Hip hyperextension is not something everyone can do right away, you need flexibility at the front, something you'll need to work on over a duration of time.

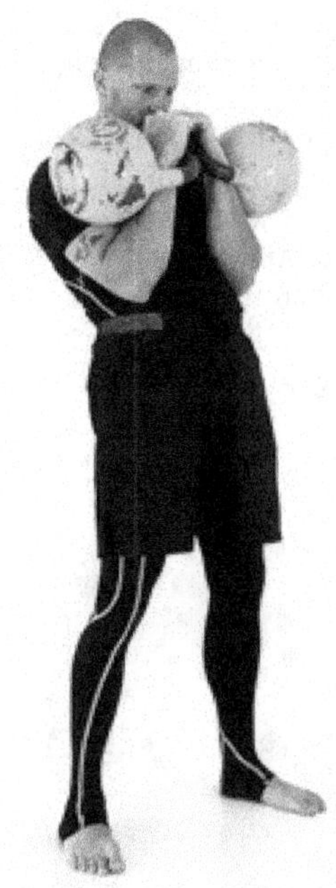

In a neutral position you'd be in extension, going further back, i.e. pulling the pelvis further back, is called hip hyperextension. But most people associate 'injury' with the word hyperextension, and its definition is:

> Hyperextension is an excessive joint movement in which the angle formed by the bones of a particular joint is opened, or straightened, beyond its normal, healthy, range of motion.

Hyper means: over; beyond; above.

Hyperextension without flexibility is indeed a cause for injury and hyperextension in joints that are not made to hyperextend is also cause for injury. Hyperextension with proper flexibility and progression is something everyone should strive for. Joints that can be hyperextended through a proper progression are:

- Hips
- Spine (back/neck)

You create hip extension by squeezing the gluteus maximus and letting the top of the femur come slightly forward, i.e. normally positioned above the ankles, now coming forward towards the toes. This action tilts the pelvis backward. On top of the pelvis is the spine, this follows along naturally—resembling back hyperextension—if you keep it positioned neutrally.

The second step is to crunch, bring the shoulders and head forward, this is done via thoracic flexion, the same action you make when performing crunches on the ground.

Racking should not be confused with back hyperextension, although back hyperextensions are also something one should be doing, and is completely safe with proper progression, it is however, not a safe nor an efficient position to rest in with heavy weights. Back hyperextension is actually the complete opposite of what a good racking position is. A good racking position is with thoracic flexion (think crunching), hip hyperextension, with knee extension, and slight ankle dorsiflexion.

Hike Back

The hike back is one of the most common movements used for starting swings, snatches, cleans, or anything that requires the bell to come from the ground and then out and up. The most common movement to perform this with is the hip hinge but a squat can also be used. The most important safety points are:

- Neutral spine
- Kettlebells come through just under or around knee height

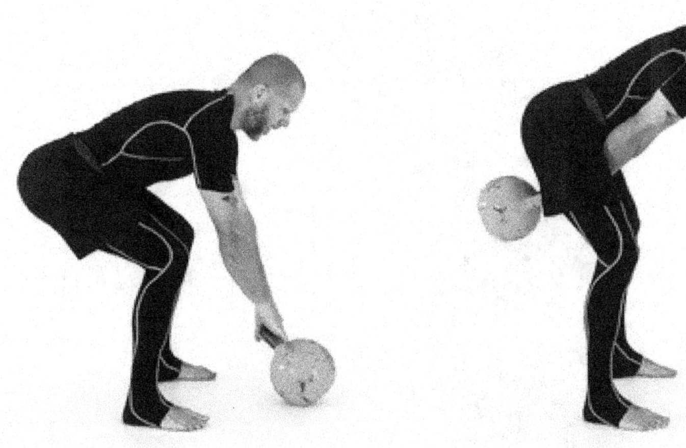

The pull should be controlled and not violent. The pull should bring the arms into a gentle connection with the body as demonstrated in the second photo above. The pull can only be safe and natural when there is enough space between you and the kettlebell, without sufficient space, it will turn into a push between the legs rather than a pull. The space required is different from person to person but as long as the same position as demonstrated in the first photo is achieved it will be safe.

Kettlebells come through just under or around knee height.

This will all vary depending on body composition but the main thing to keep in mind is to keep the shoulders above the hips with a neutral spine. Direct the weights to the back rather than low to the ground, low to the ground would mean a pull up is required, whereas far back would give you momentum from the kettlebells using gravity. This is not to say that performing this with a pull is bad, it can be good if its what your goal requires, but in general this movement is performed to take advantage of momentum.

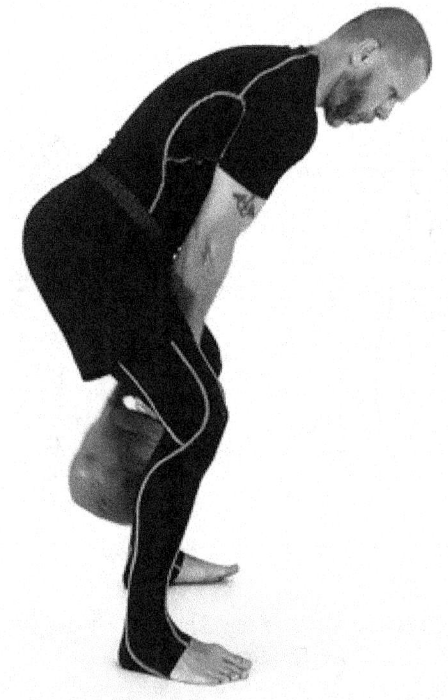

The hike back can be performed with one or two kettlebells, and with one or two arms. When using two kettlebells you will need to use a wider stance but at the same time making sure the knees don't buckle out.

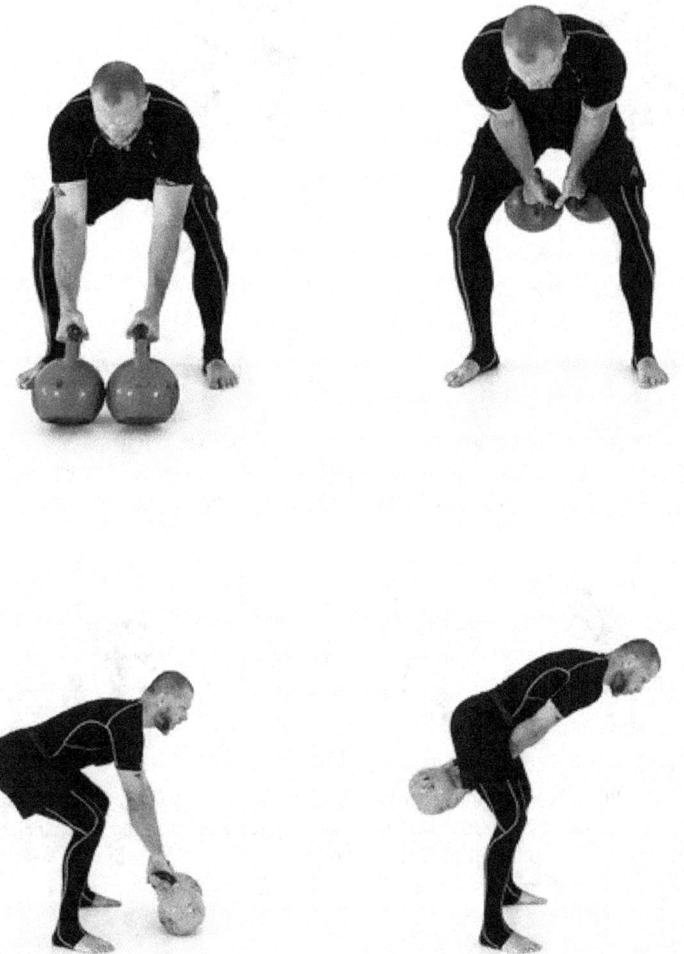

Always create some tension between you and the weight before pulling. See the first photo.

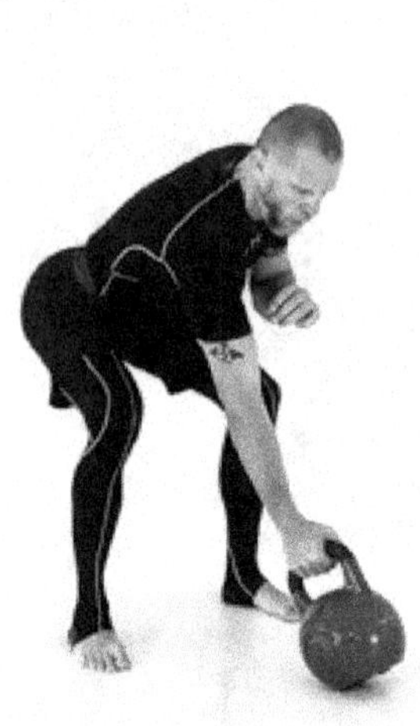 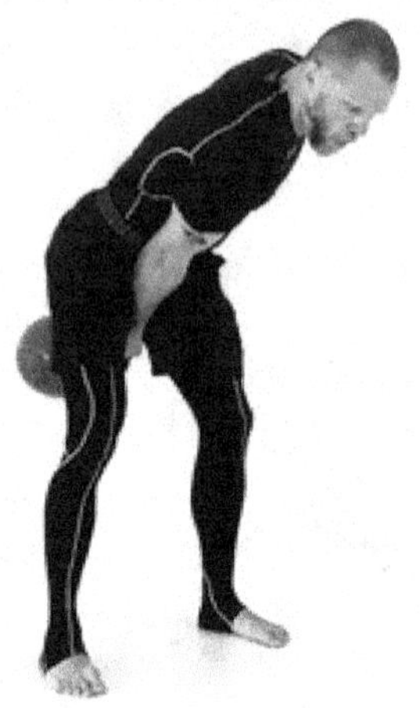

The hike back is commonly part of or used to transition into another exercise, but it can just as well be used as an exercise on its own, and I personally use it to break down the kettlebell swing and perfect the position into which the backswing should end. This looks as following.

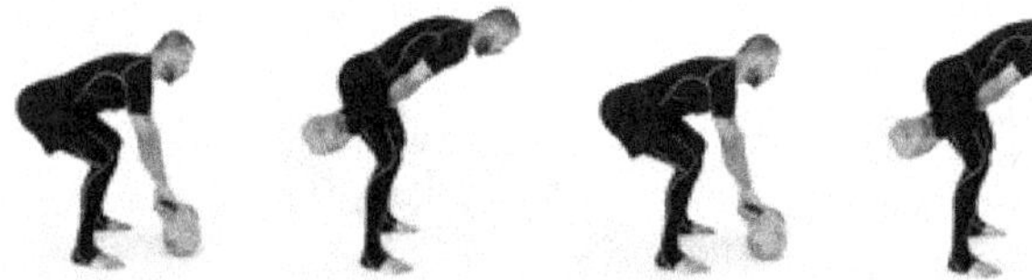

Apart from it teaching the athlete what the end of the backswing should feel like, it also engrains the position for the first part of starting a swing. The main areas worked here are the posterior chain muscles and the quadriceps. For the pull, all muscles responsible for shoulder extension are used. There is minimal movement when it comes to hip or knee extension, hence, this is mostly isometric apart from the pull.

Counterbalance

Looking at the dictionary for the word *counterbalance*:

- a weight that balances another weight.

- a factor having the opposite effect to that of another and so preventing it from exercising a disproportionate influence.

The following photos are a great example of good counterbalance during the drop from the rack. As the weights fall forward the upper body comes back and away from the weights which creates an even counterbalance to prevent disproportionate load on the lower back.

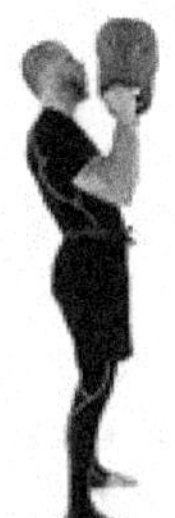 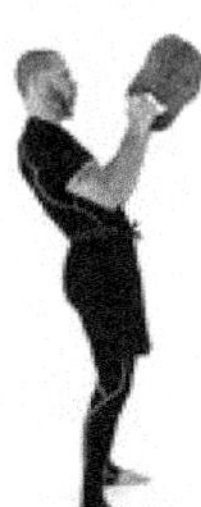 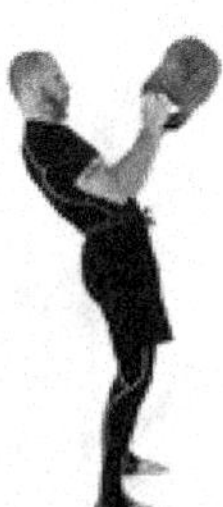 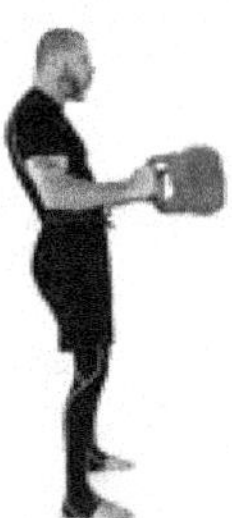

The amount of counterbalance required increases with the amount of weight used, the heavier the weight the more one needs to work on counterbalancing during movements. There are several areas through which counterbalance can be created:

- Ankles (plantar flexion)
- Knees (flexion)
- Hips (hyperextension)
- Thoracic spine (hyperextension)

Drop

Whether you're dropping the weight from racking or overhead, you should never follow the kettlebell. What this means is, as soon as you initiate the drop, don't bend at the hips too, if you're bending at the hips the moment the weight drops (comes forward) then you're compromising your lower back, you're putting unnecessary pressure/stress on it. With the drop from rack you want to be in extension or even hyperextension, at the point the bell is around/below the hip area which all depends on whether the arm is straight or not, if it's not, don't come out of extension yet. The same applies to the full drop from overhead, however, due to the kettlebell being further away from the body, the arm will be extended sooner, hence, the follow-through happens sooner than with the drop from the rack.

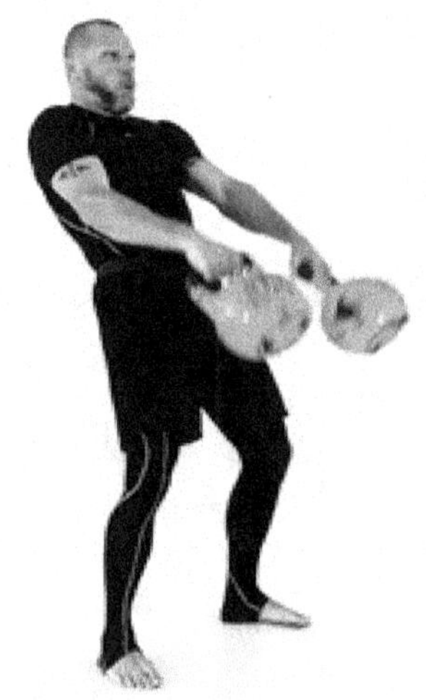

More information on this topic can be found under the clean and swing.

A good example of the drop can be seen in slow-motion in this video go.cavemantraining.com/kbe-vid-001

Rack/Racking

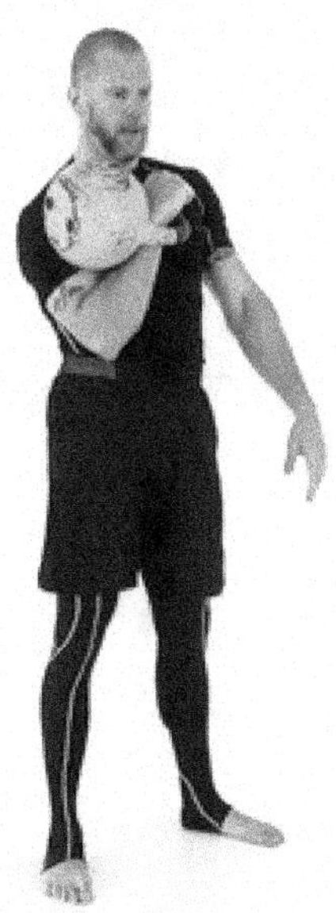

Dot points:

- Kettlebell racking happens after you clean a kettlebell

- The rack can be a resting or transitional position

- A bad racking position can burn out the shoulders or affect the forearm

- With a transitional rack your elbow should be tucked/pulled into your obliques/ribs

- Use your latissimus dorsi to pull the elbow/arm in

- Rest the bell on the biceps and forearm

- A little bit of space at the bottom of the elbow is ok for a transitional rack

- Place the elbow on the ilium to transfer power for jerking or push pressing

- For resting you want to rest the elbow on the ilium

- During sport/endurance/high volume reps you want to use a good rack to be able to rest with the bell up

- A disconnected arm means shoulder flexion which means additional and unnecessary work

- Let the weight rest on your skeletal system and not your muscular system

- Although it might look like it's bad for the lumbar there is actually no movement in the lumbar

- All range is created through hip hyperextension and extension plus flexion in the thoracic

- A good rack requires flexibility in the hips and thoracic

- Squeeze the gluteus maximus to pull the top of the pelvis back

- Let the top of the femur come slightly forward

- Getting better range in the hip flexors takes time

- Hip hyperextension and crunch

- A rounded back is not a problem because we're not pressing

- You want to rack with just enough contraction to obtain a good posture

- The weight naturally wants to fall away from the body which requires work to pull in

- Make space to let the weight rest on/above the legs

- A cradle rack is an option for females with larger breasts

- The rack is a position you need to learn properly

Kettlebell Exercises

A kettlebell exercise, in effect, is a bodyweight exercise to which resistance is added in the form of a kettlebell. An exercise has variations. Several exercises strung together become a combo (combination). In this encyclopedia of kettlebell exercises I will cover the purest form of an exercise, variations, and some combinations as a bonus.

Kettlebell Press

The press can be split into two categories horizontal and vertical. Vertical is where the torso is positioned vertical, i.e. standing or seated, and horizontal is where the torso is positioned horizontal, i.e. laying down.

The vertical press is to target the shoulder and the horizontal press is to target the chest more.

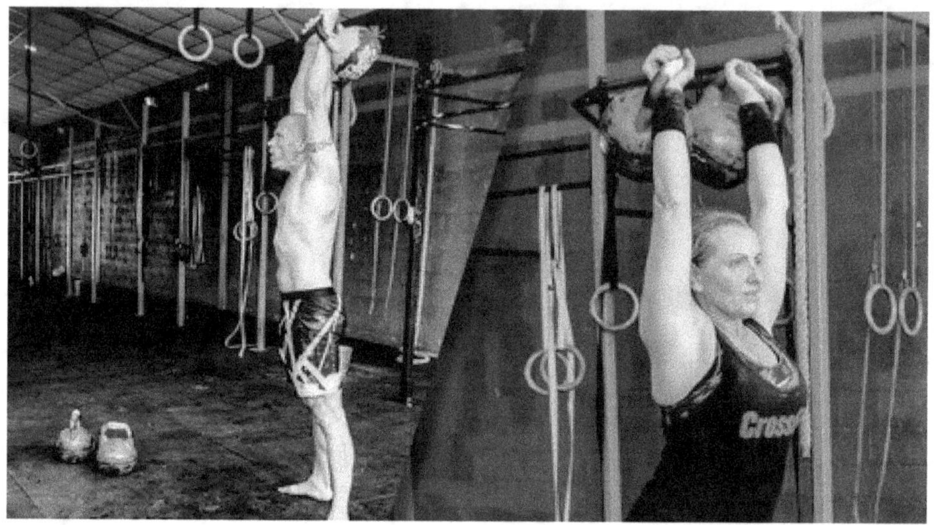

Front Press

AKA: Shoulder press, overhead press

The overhead press is usually looked at as just a shoulder exercise but there is so much more to it. A good press requires a good base, this means strength and stability from the shoulders down as well as the shoulders. The deltoids are the prime movers but the triceps also come into play for the elbow extension, which is the part that straightens the arm and keeps it straight once overhead.

The front press or often referred to as the strict press is a shoulder press where the weight stays at the front during the press overhead. The prime mover is the deltoid but the position of the kettlebell dictates what part of the deltoid is worked the most. With the front press, it is the anterior (front) of the deltoid.

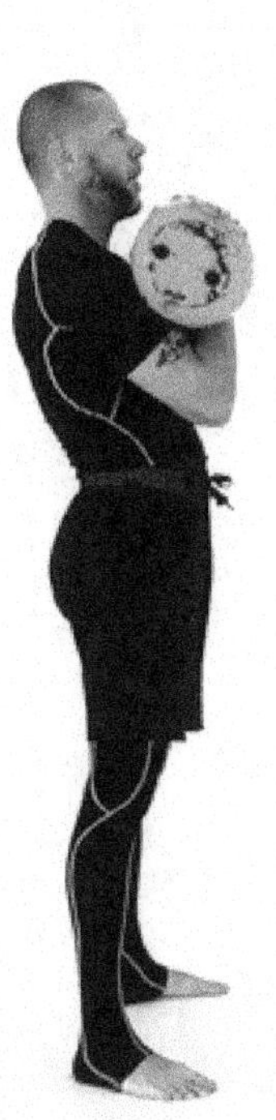

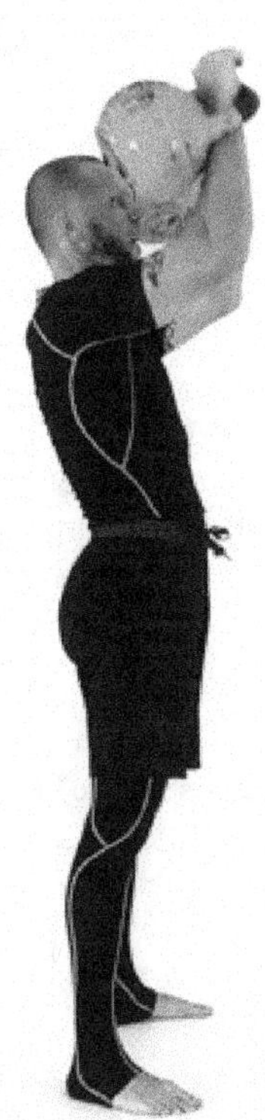

Getting back to 'strict' as this press often is referred to, strict does not define anything about the press other than the movement with which the press is performed, without momentum, i.e. no help from the legs, thoracic, or other body parts other than the shoulders.

The easiest and most efficient—I repeat, efficient is not always what we want in training—way to press is the shortest path to the end destination, meaning to press back and up at the same time. You can also press up first and then back which provides the greatest tension on the deltoid. The further away the kettlebells are from being above the deltoid during the press the more tension it provides.

The double kettlebell press provides a more overall load on the body whereas the single-arm press provides more benefit to the obliques.

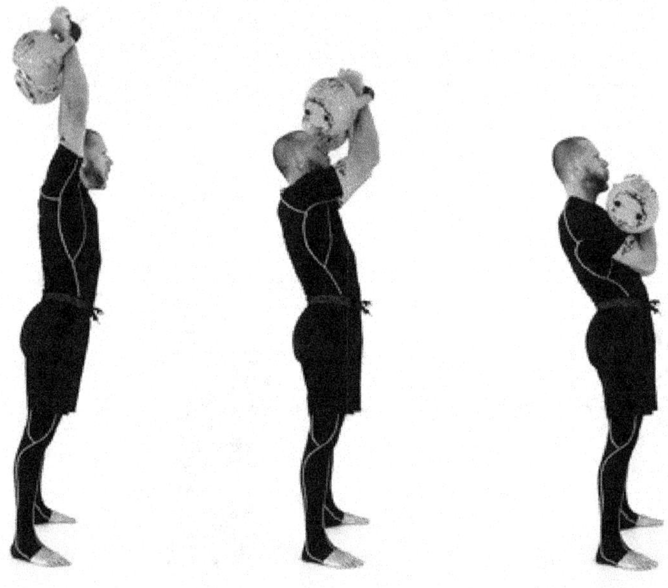

The following sequence shows how to clean the kettlebells for the front press but can also be used as a combo in workouts.

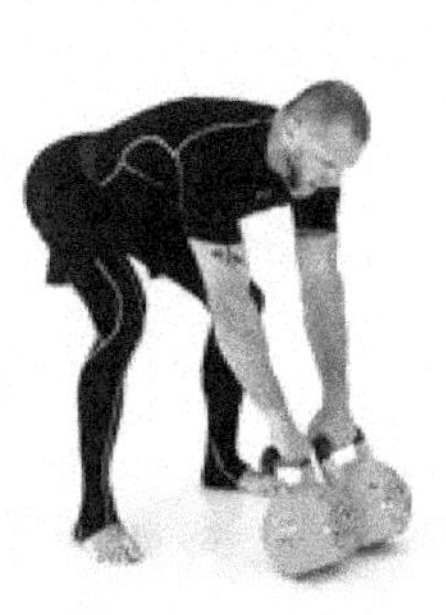 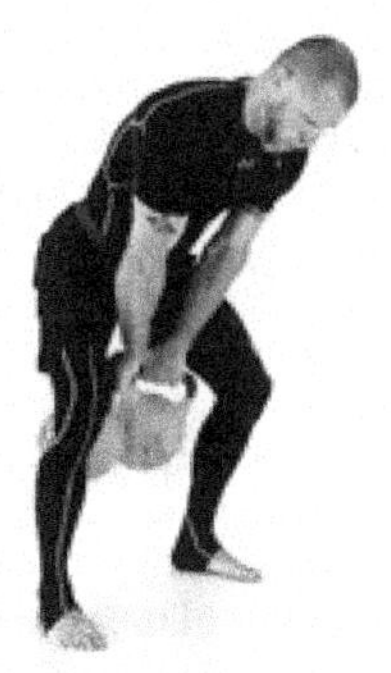 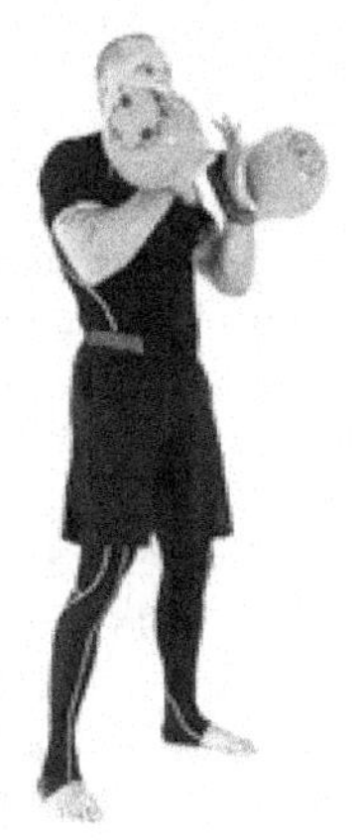

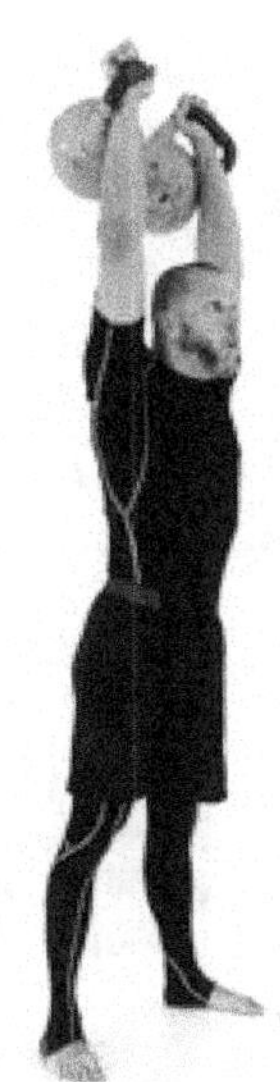

Dot points:

- Before you can press you will need to clean and rack
- Create tension before you press and lock everything out so not to lose power
- Tension and locking out creates a stable base to press from but also recruits more muscles

- Protect your lower back through gluteus maximus contraction (and hamstrings)
- As the bell comes overhead you're moving underneath it
- You want to end up directly under the kettlebell
- It's ok to work on overhead range with a lightweight
- The triceps lock out the elbow
- Keep the shoulder safe through lat engagement and pulling the scapulae slightly down
- Once overhead let the weight rest on the skeletal system but keep pressing up
- Obtain a good overhead lockout on each rep
- Work on the full range for mobility and flexibility
- Full range means longer under tension which is good for strength
- Keep the elbow under the weight during the press

Bonus videos:
- 50+ Kettlebell Press Exercises go.cavemantraining.com/kbe-vid-68
- Military Press VS Front Press go.cavemantraining.com/kbe-vid-69
- Combo Dead Swing Clean, Squat, And Press go.cavemantraining.com/kbe-vid-70
- The Difference Between Front And Side Shoulder Press go.cavemantraining.com/kbe-vid-71

Bonus workouts:
- The SIXPRESS Kettlebell Combo For Strong Shoulders + Core go.cavemantraining.com/kbe-vid-72
- WOD "NotDoneYet2.0" Insanely Good go.cavemantraining.com/kbe-vid-73
- THE BIG FOUR: Kettlebell Strength Workout go.cavemantraining.com/kbe-vid-74

Open Palm Grip

Using different grips with the press will create different stability challenges, which is a good thing if you want to train and improve stability. Improvement in stability will shine through as improvement in your press and pressing strength.

The open palm grip places the weight in the palm and adds stability challenges during the press. The most instability provided by a grip is the bottoms-up grip.

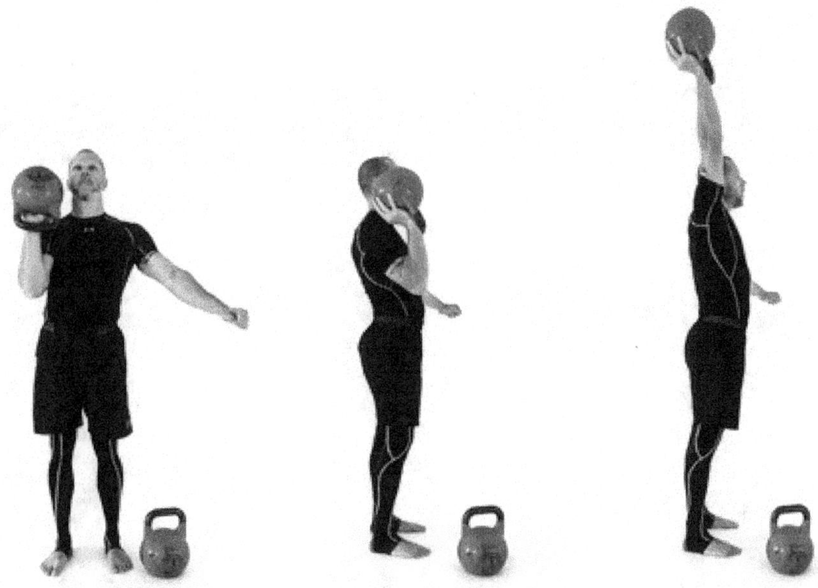

When using one kettlebell you can place the bell in your palm with the other hand or use an open palm clean. When working with two kettlebells you are forced to use the open palm clean.

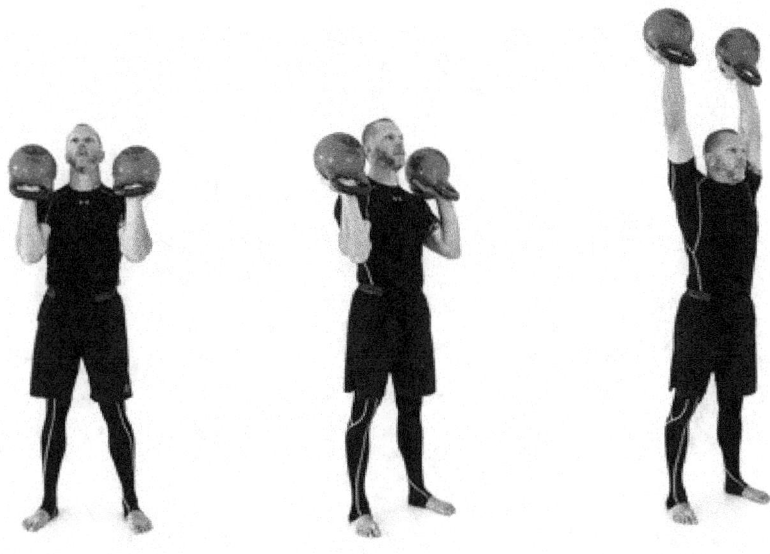

Waiters Grip

The waiters grip is the next step up in creating instability. This grip requires more wrist strength as there is more hyperextension than there is with the open palm grip. Before you attempt this exercise you should make sure you have the appropriate flexibility and use the correct weight. Training the wrist is good and often overlooked, hence, an area prone to injury when going too fast too soon.

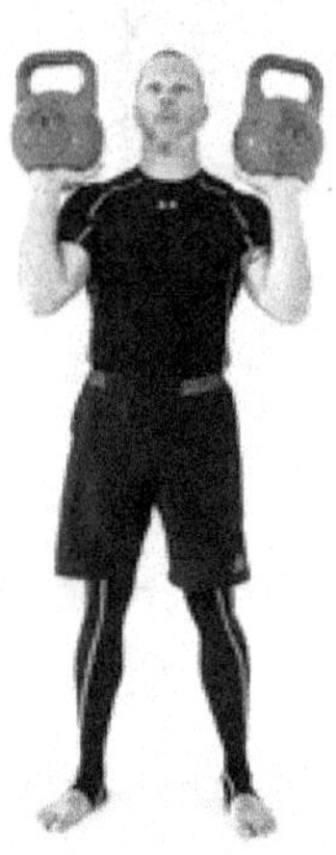 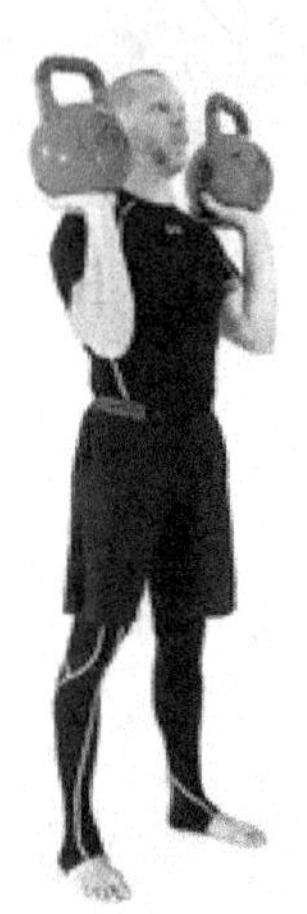 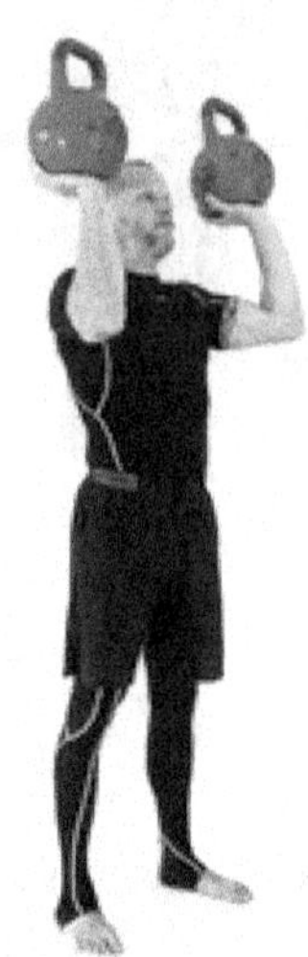

The waiters clean just like the open palm clean is a juggling exercise.

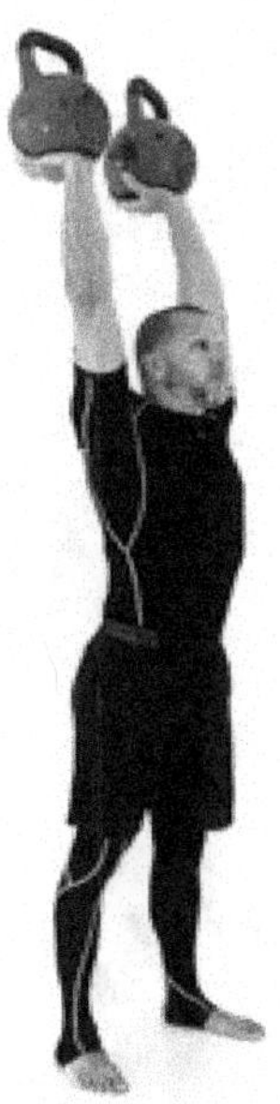

Alternating Press

The alternating press is performed with two kettlebells. The press is initiated on one side while the other remains racked and waiting for the overhead kettlebell to return into racking before it is pressed up while the other waits in racking position.

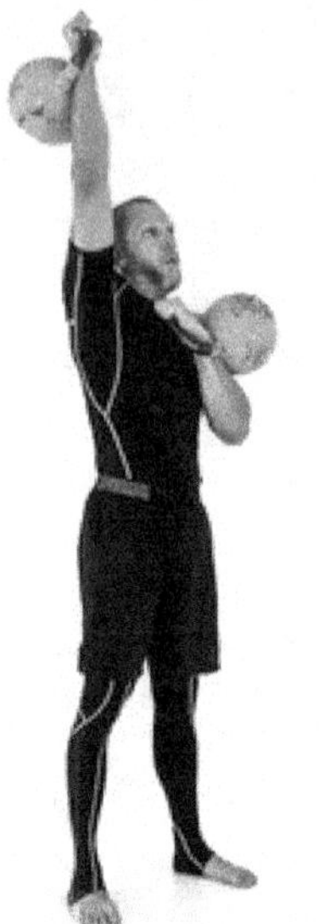 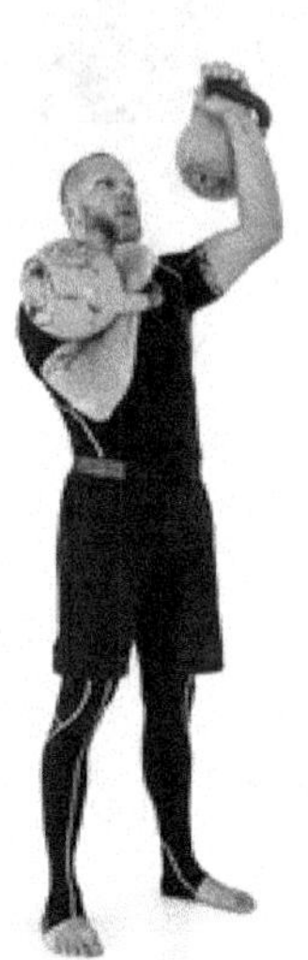 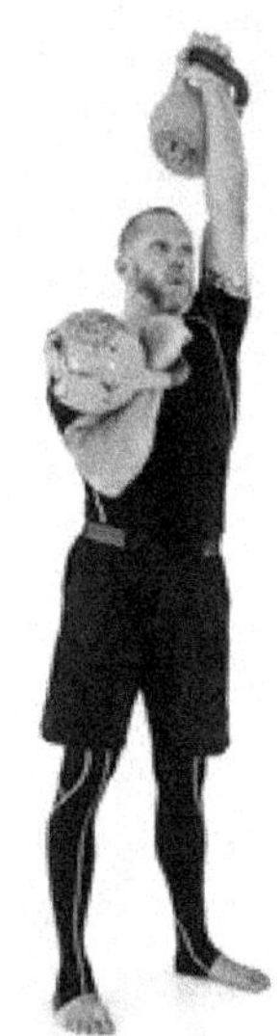

Bent Press

The bent press is one of these exercises that were the staple of old-time strongmen such as Eugen Sandow, Arthur Saxon, and Louis Cyr. It's not a very popular exercise anymore but at Cavemantraining we're working on bringing it back as it's an exercise everyone should be incorporating in their training, it's awesome for so many things.

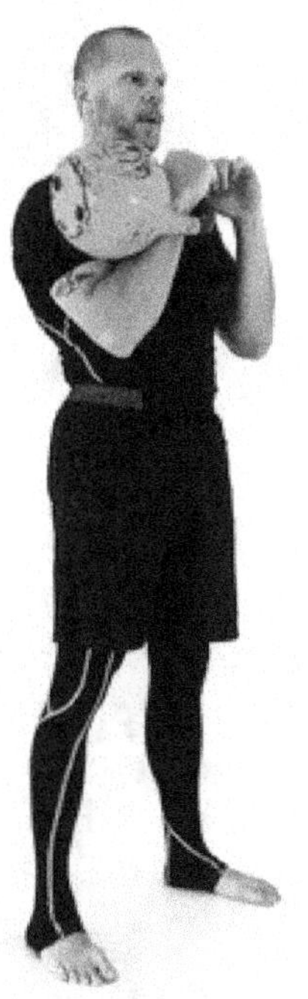
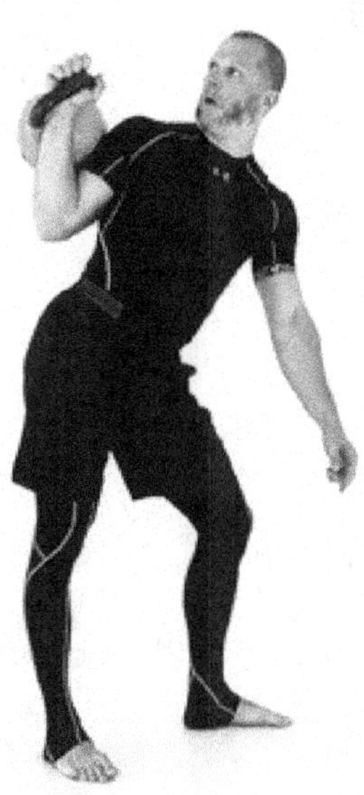

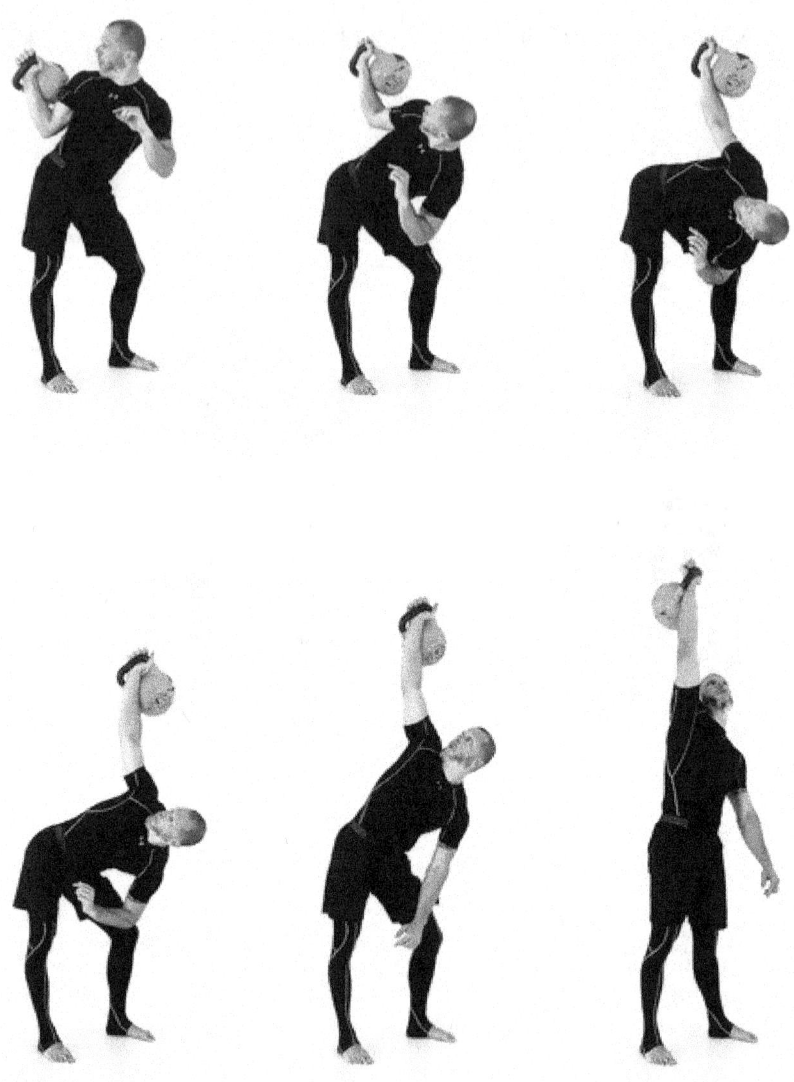

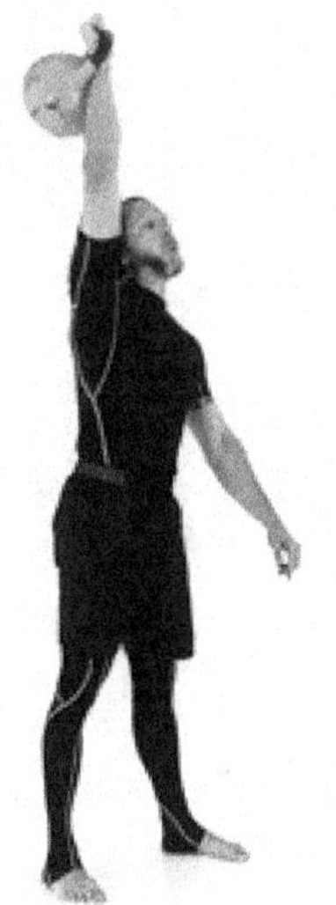
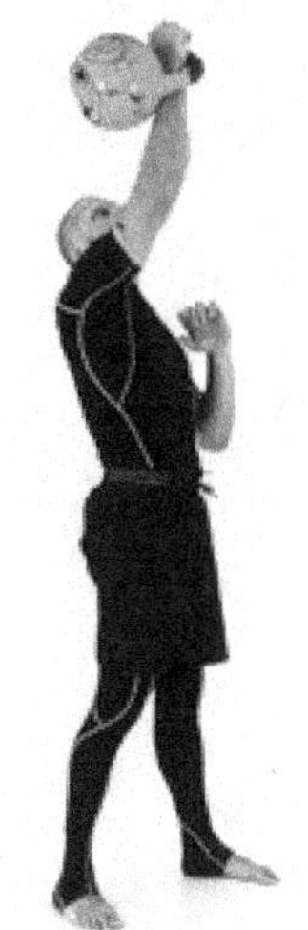
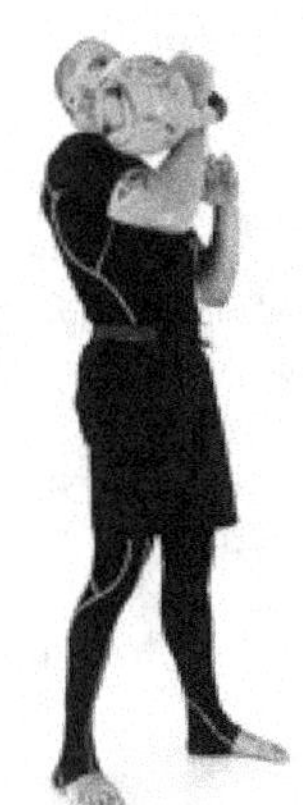
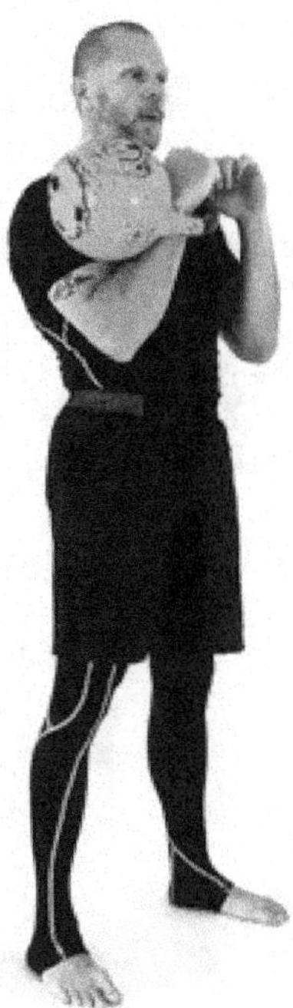

Why:

- Thoracic mobility
- Flexibility
- Core strength
- Shoulder mobility
- Shoulder strength
- Improved posture
- Injury prevention
- Kyphosis prevention (rounding of the back)
- Improved breathing
- Stability and so much more

It's also great to get heavier weight overhead and focus on the down-phase of the overhead position, i.e. increase your pressing strength.

Unlike the name suggests, it's not a press, in summary, is performed as follows:

1. Rack
2. Rotate
3. Pull
4. Bent
5. Come under
6. Lock out
7. Come up
8. Shoulder rotation
9. Neutral stance
10. Rack and repeat

One can come under the weight in different ways, one leg locked other bent or bending both knees and turn it more into a squat under.

This awesome exercise requires progression, you will need to work on your flexibility first, hamstrings especially, you'll need to work on shoulders, work on rotation with just bodyweight, work on the movement without weight, then slowly increase the weight over time.

Minimum requirements:

- Thoracic rotation 35°
- Hip flexion 90°
- External shoulder rotation 35°

Progression:
- Hip hinge
- Thoracic rotation
- Shoulder internal and external rotation
- Breaking down the movements
- Perfect the full bodyweight movement

- Add lightweight
- Increase reps
- Increase weight

Breaking down the movements

After all other requirements are met and you've come to the point of breaking down the movement pattern, that works as follows.

Drill 1. Rotation and arm placement:

- Repeat thoracic rotation with one arm bent
- Active lat to keep pulling the elbow down throughout the movement
- Follow the hand with your eyesight
- Try and keep the hips as straight as possible
- Keep the forearm vertical
- Repeat

Drill 2. Coming under the weight:

- Continue at the extend of drill 1
- Bring the non-working arm to the chest and keep it there
- Hip hinge or squat to bring the hips and shoulders down
- Keep the hand at the same level throughout the movement
- Push yourself away from the hand till full elbow extension
- Do not press the hand up
- Repeat

If you need support then you can use the elbow of the non-working arm to press into the thigh. Pressing into the thigh will relieve tension on the back/abs. You can also use the hand on the non-working arm to pull on the thigh for support, this would be opposite of pressing the elbow into the thigh of the other leg.

Drill 3. Coming up:

- Continue at the extend of drill 2
- Keep the arm up throughout the drill
- Come into the bottom position and back up
- Focus on the shoulder rotation that happens during the movement
- Come into a full neutral standing position with the arm overhead

5 reps per drill on each side will be good, but you should pick a number of reps that feels good for you. Work for 5 minutes, rest, and repeat at 4 times to understand the movement.

After having drilled all the movements you put them all together and act like you're working with a real weight. I should note that sometimes the drilling becomes easier when you do have some added weight even if as low as 4 or 8kg, and sometimes the whole movement improves once you start adding real weight, 12kg, 16kg and up.

     Kettlebell Exercise Encyclopedia VOL. 3   Taco Fleur

When working with heavier weights you can implement the double-handed clean.

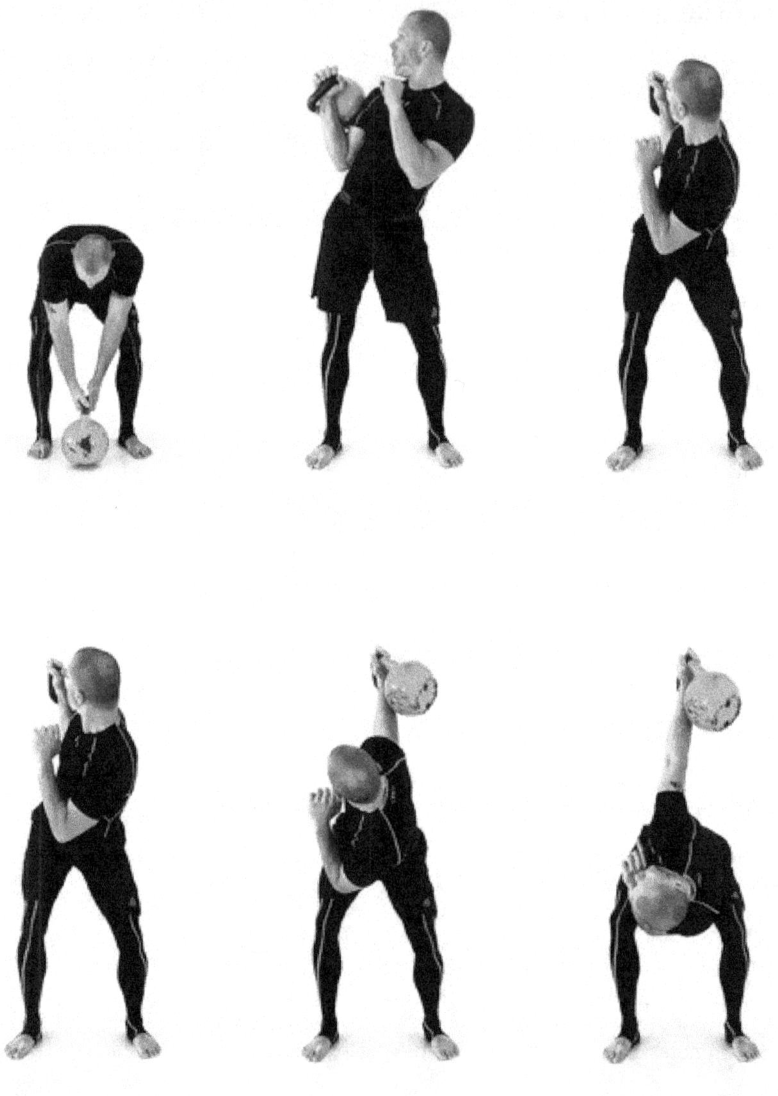

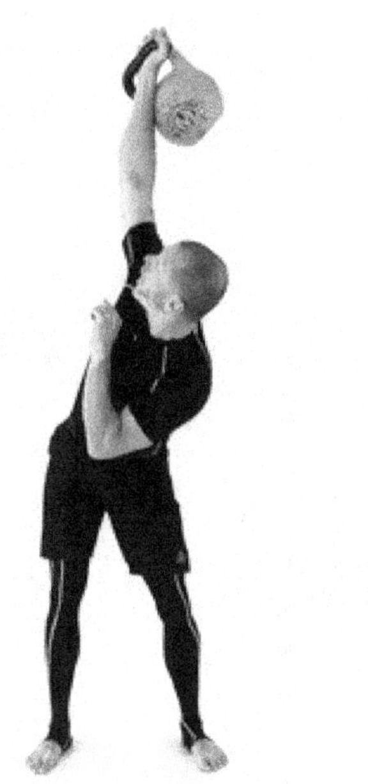 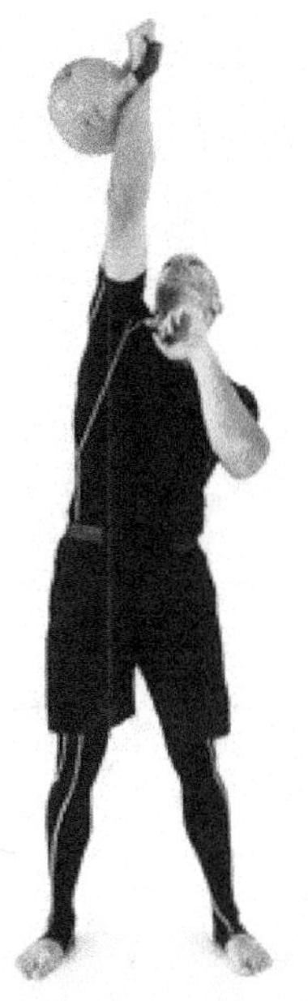 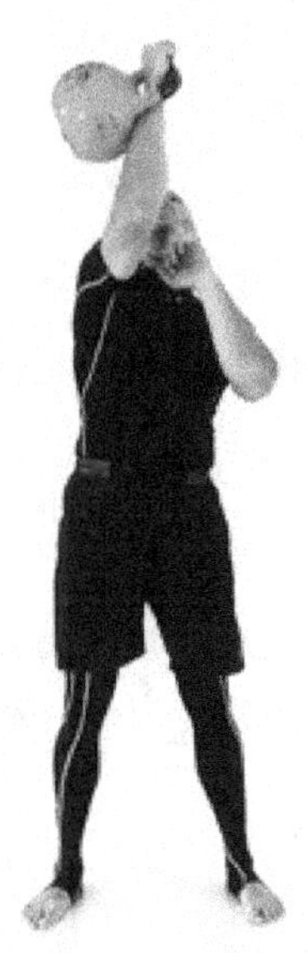

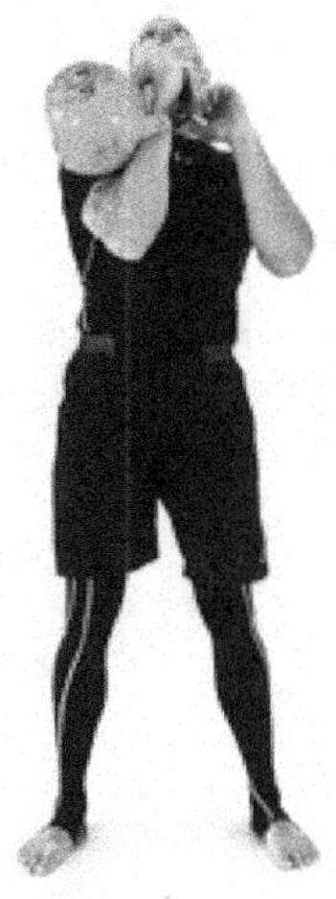

The bent press is a great exercise to everything in your midsection, the less support you give your core the harder it needs to work. Once you're using a heavier weight or even when you're just starting out you can place the non-working hand on the thigh for support and assistance through triceps and shoulder extension.

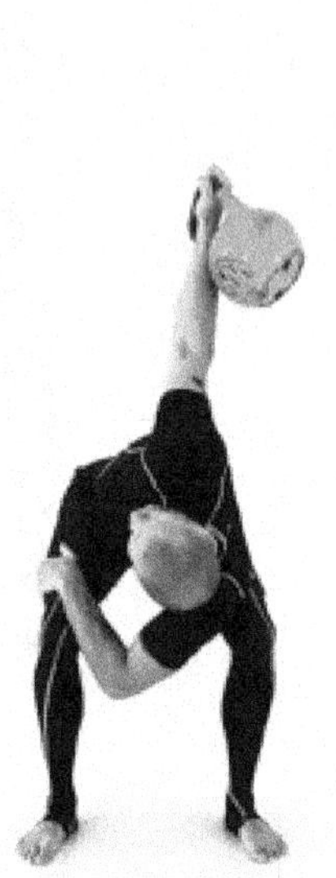 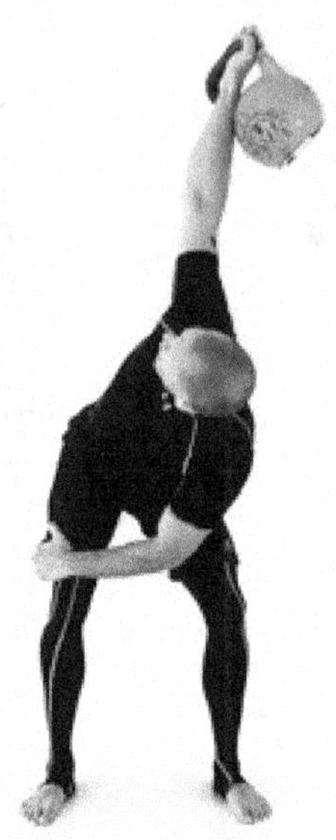

Bonus videos:
- Kettlebell Bent Press go.cavemantraining.com/kbe-vid-75
- Kneeling Bent Press For Mobility go.cavemantraining.com/kbe-vid-76
- Kettlebell Bent Press go.cavemantraining.com/kbe-vid-77
- 80kg Bent Press By Oliver Quinn go.cavemantraining.com/kbe-vid-78
- Workout With Bent Press Deadlift Variation go.cavemantraining.com/kbe-vid-79

Bonus workouts:
- The SIXPRESS Kettlebell Combo go.cavemantraining.com/kbe-vid-80

Bent Side Press

This variation of the press is another one of those unconventional exercises that you hardly see performed anymore. I believe that is because the benefits of the exercise were lost over time and thus seen as a useless exercise, it's not. If you perform this right and understand the benefits you should reap from it then you'll start to love it.

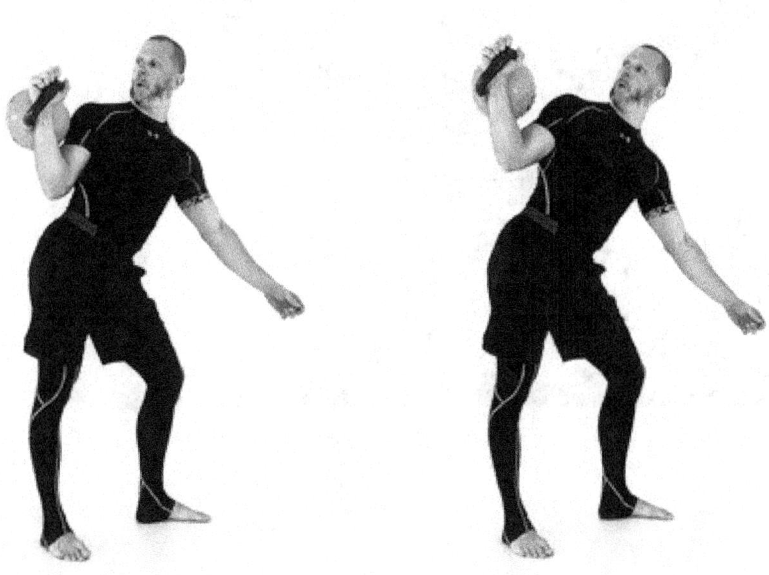

The benefits are latissimus dorsi, shoulders, and core or rather the muscles that keep the spine straight and protect it. Due to the angle of the press, it targets the side deltoid and produces a force on the spine from an angle it normally does not receive any. This is a great benefit. As you're pressing up to the side the force wants to laterally flex the spine the left (see photo), this force has to be resisted which is a good thing to train the muscles.

Unlike most shoulder press variations, this variation does not press up but to the side, when you're at the end of the press and you would keep your arm at the endpoint of the press and stand up straight, the arm would be in the same position as in an Iron Cross (see photo).

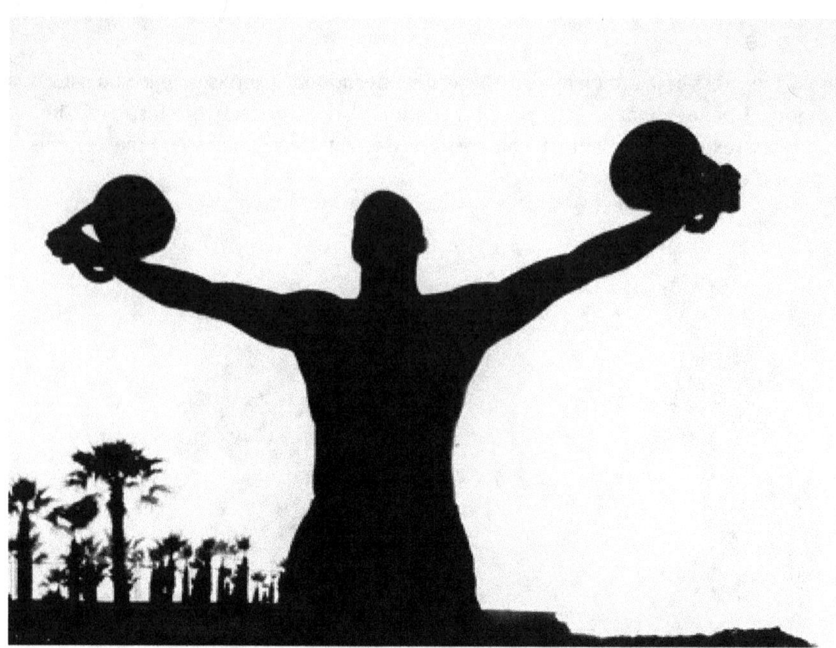

Kettlebell Iron Cross.

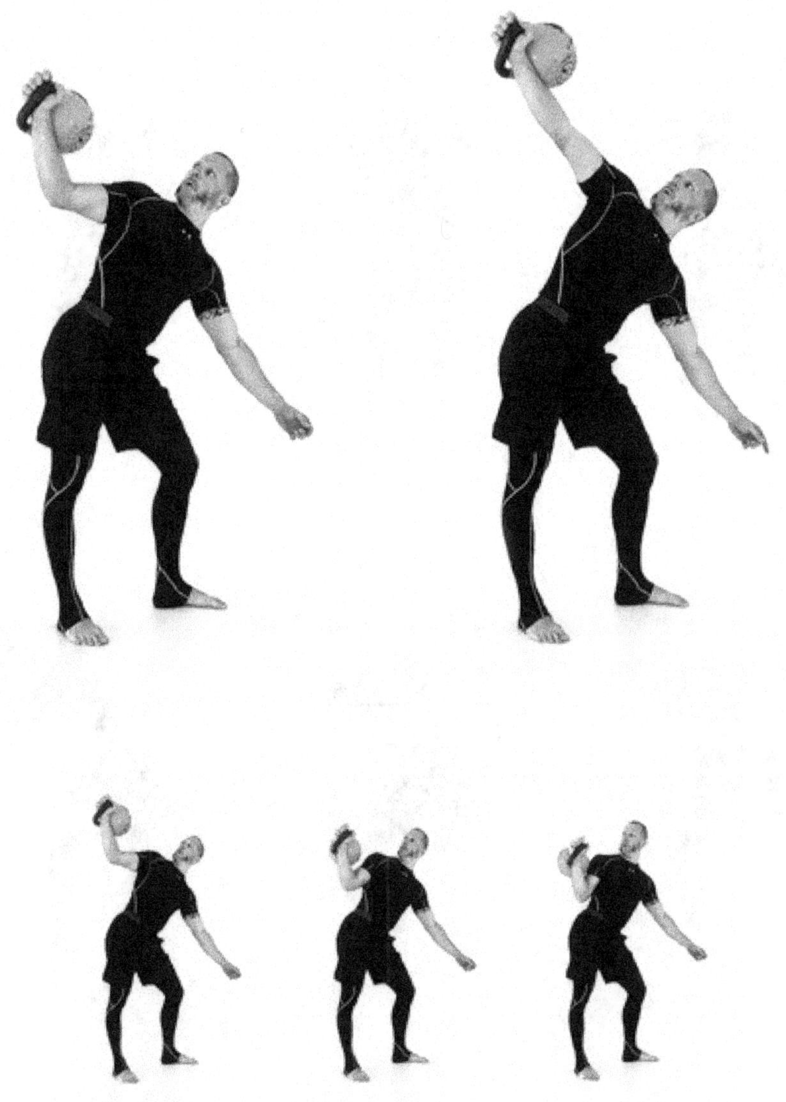

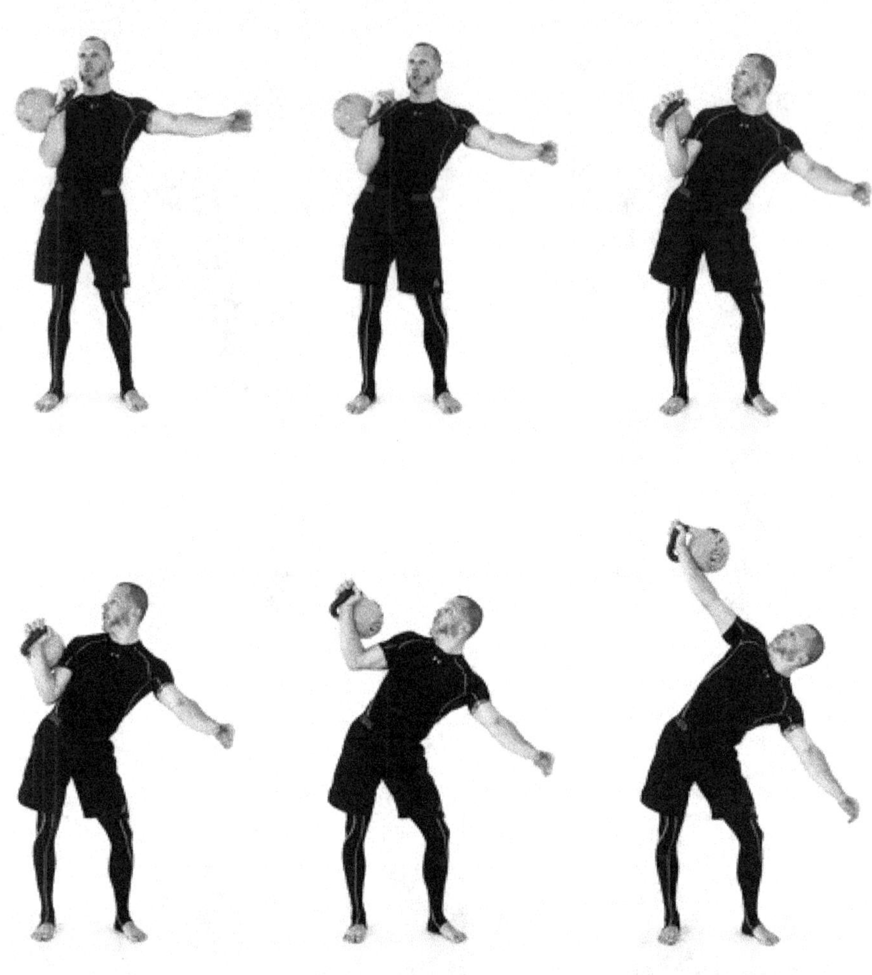

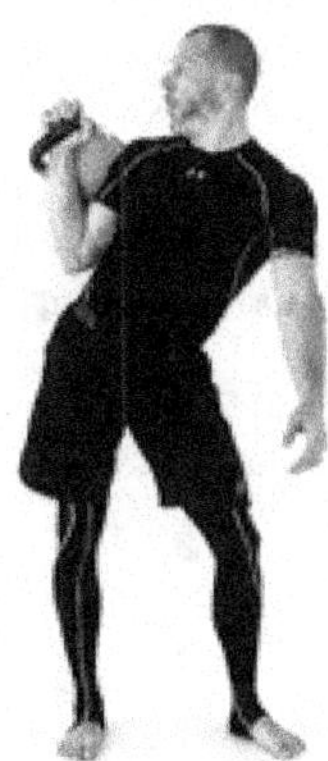

When you perform this exercise you not only already need some deltoid strength but core strength as well, in fact, whether you'll be able to comfortably do this exercise will depend on your core strength and flexibility.

To perform:

- Start in racking position
- Push the hip to one side
- Bend the knee of the side you're pushing away from
- Keep the knee straight on the side you're pushing into
- Externally rotate the shoulder
- Pull the elbow toward the hip
- Depending on your flexibility the elbow can be on the side or slightly behind
- Keep the forearm close to vertical at the start
- Keep the spine straight
- Brace all the muscles around the spine for the force to come
- Start pressing up and laterally out
- Keep the press lateral
- Pause at the end position
- Control the movement
- Return to starting position

Bonus videos:
* Bent Side Press Bottoms Up go.cavemantraining.com/kbe-vid-81

Bonus workouts:
* The SIXPRESS Kettlebell Combo go.cavemantraining.com/kbe-vid-82
* The Grinding Warrior Workout go.cavemantraining.com/kbe-vid-83

Floor Press

The floor press is a press variation where you're laying horizontally on the floor while pressing. When placing your feet flat on the ground in line with the hips gives you more stability, the wider you go with the feet outside the hips the more stability you create. Doing the opposite, bringing the feet together or leg flat and together will remove stability, thus creating instability, depending on your goal or state of conditioning, instability might what you need for the added challenge.

Each of the following press variations ends up with the hands being directly above the shoulder and triceps locking out the elbows. At the start of each press you want the hands to be placed above the elbows, forearm vertical for maximum range and benefits. Following are variations of the floor press.

Triceps Press

The elbows are shaving the ribs or as close to them as your flexibility allows.

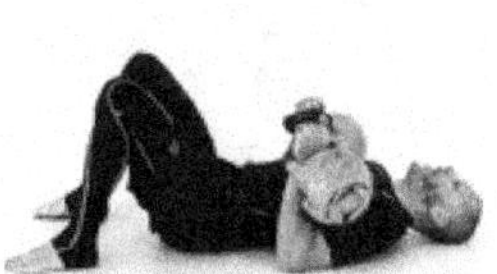 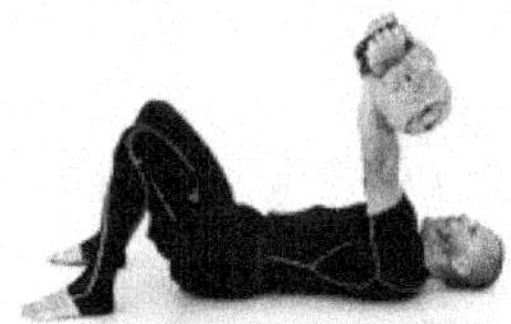

Hybrid Floor Press

There is a 45 degree angle between the elbows and ribs.

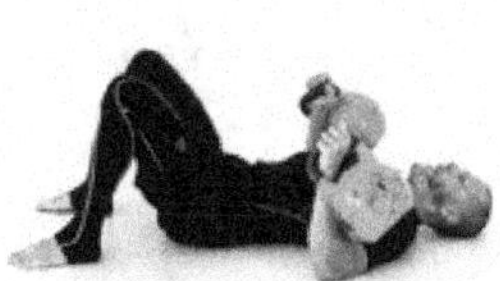 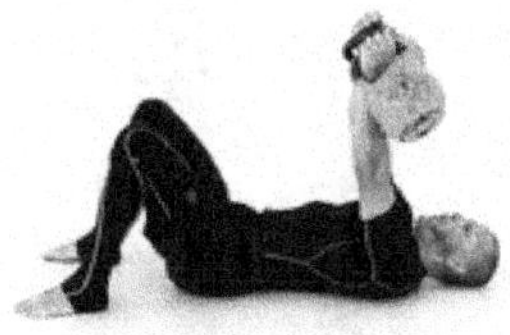

Chest Press

There is a 90 degree angle between the elbows and ribs. The focus of this floor press is on the chest.

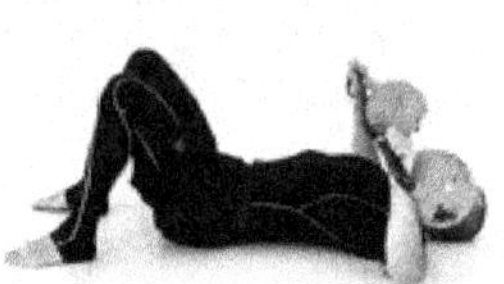 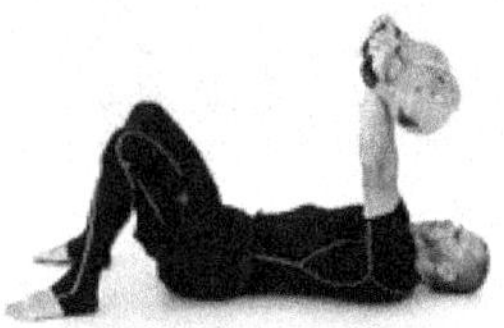

Bonus videos:
Kettlebell Exercise: Chest Press Unilateral go.cavemantraining.com/kbe-vid-84
10+ Kettlebell Chest Exercises go.cavemantraining.com/kbe-vid-85
Chest Press Unilateral go.cavemantraining.com/kbe-vid-86

Bonus workouts:
THE BIG FOUR: Kettlebell Strength Workout go.cavemantraining.com/kbe-vid-87

Alternating Chest Press

The alternating chest press is where one kettlebell waits for the other to return before pressing. You can vary the angle worked in. Demonstrated is the alternating chest press (90 degree angle).

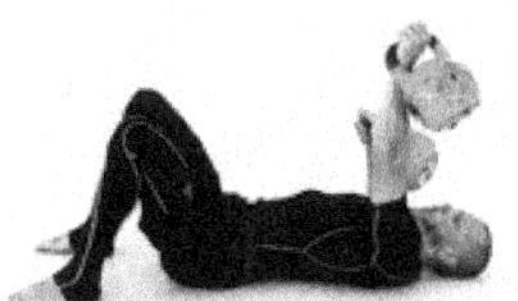 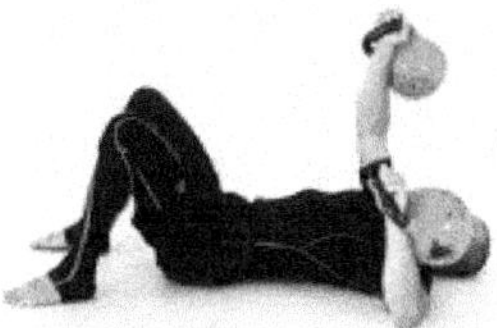

Bridging Chest Press

Bringing will add additional muscle groups to the exercise, namely the hamstrings, gastrocnemius, and other muscles, but it also adds additional shoulder extension, this is not additional range but putting your shoulder extension to the test, hence, great if it's an area you need to work on. Lifting one leg off the floor will add more load on one leg but also requires more hip stability.

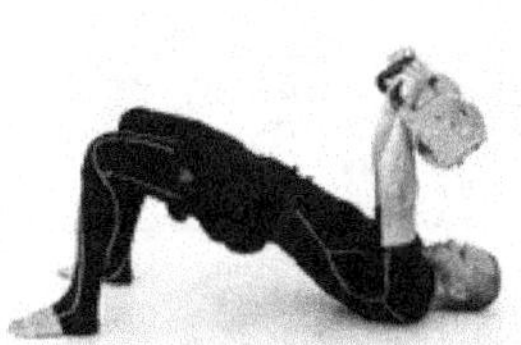 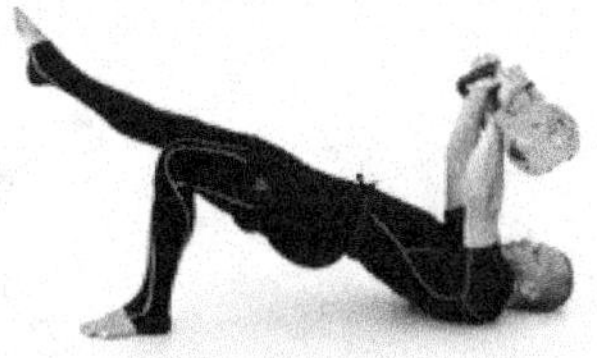

Floor Crush Grip Press

This variation of the floor press is not about making the press easier because you're using two arms and one kettlebell, it's about the crushing you need to actively perform during the press, this engages the pectorals and adds a new dimension to the press. You can also flare the elbows out a bit to try and find that angle which works best for you and hits the spot. You can hold the bell without crushing it, but the point is that you do crush it to get maximum benefit.

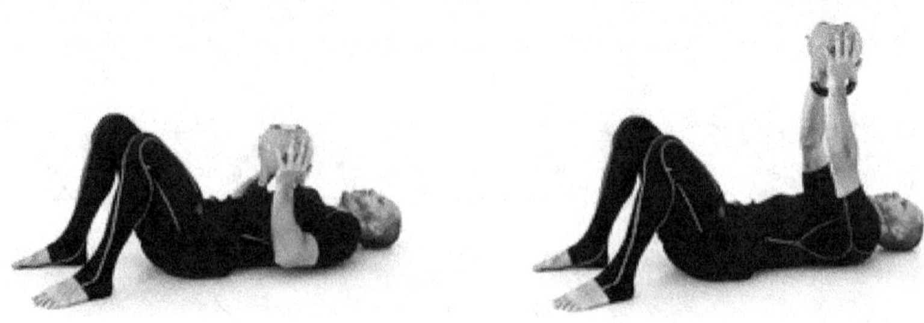

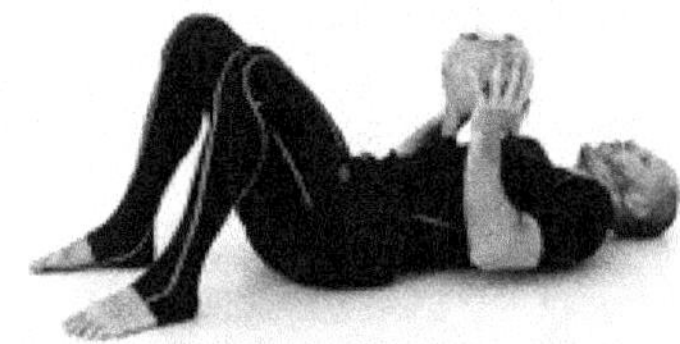

You can also vary the position of the kettlebell if you feel the handle is in the way.

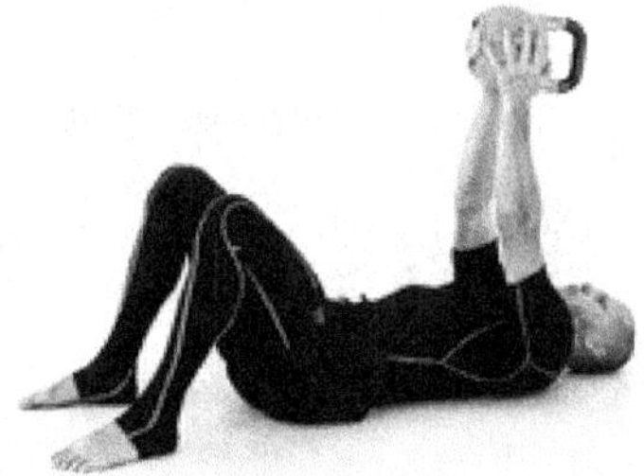

Push Press

The push press is half powered by the legs and half by the shoulder(s). While in racking, the knees flex and rapidly extend while driving into and keeping the heels on the floor. The push press is the progression to the jerk. On that note, the jerk is not a press.

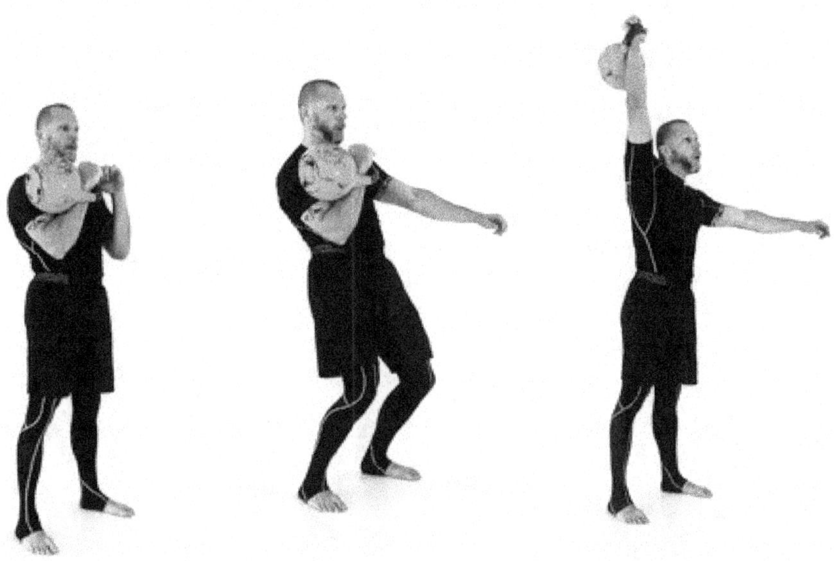

Unwillingly those who are fatigued and have a large number of shoulder presses programmed for them will turn them into a push press, i.e. they start using momentum from their lower body to get the weight overhead.

To perform:

1. Stand in a neutral stance

2. Good racking position

3. Pull the knees forward

4. Ankle dorsiflexion paired with hip flexion to push the knees forward

5. Immediately pull the knees back

6. Keep the feet flat

7. Propel the weight up

8. Press out

9. Finish with a good overhead lockout

From overhead, you can drop into racking position or you can work on the eccentric phase and control the down phase. How you want to bring it down depends on what you're working for. You might want to bring a heavier kettlebell than you can strict press overhead and then work on the negative phase, or if you're working for AMRAP then you want to drop into racking position. Whether you dampen the impact with by coming on the balls of the feet to meet the kettlebell(s) and reduce the impact all depends on the amount of weight.

Before learning the jerk you would learn to push press.

Bonus videos:
- The Difference Between Clean And Press/Push Press/Jerk go.cavemantraining.com/kbe-vid-88
- Kettlebell Combo: Hang Clean Push Press go.cavemantraining.com/kbe-vid-89

Jerk

The jerk is listed under the press but let me point out straight away that it's not a press. The weight is pushed up with the legs and then you come under. The jerk, however, is a great exercise for many things, one being to get heavier weight overhead than you can press, in turn, this helps you with pressing heavier or improve other attributes that improve your press.

The first part of the jerk is a push press that's not pressed out. Immediately after the push there is the second dip which is to come under the weight (photo 3) with the arm locked out. From there the next position is coming into full extension with the arm still overhead. The weight is then dropped into racking position and another jerk is performed.

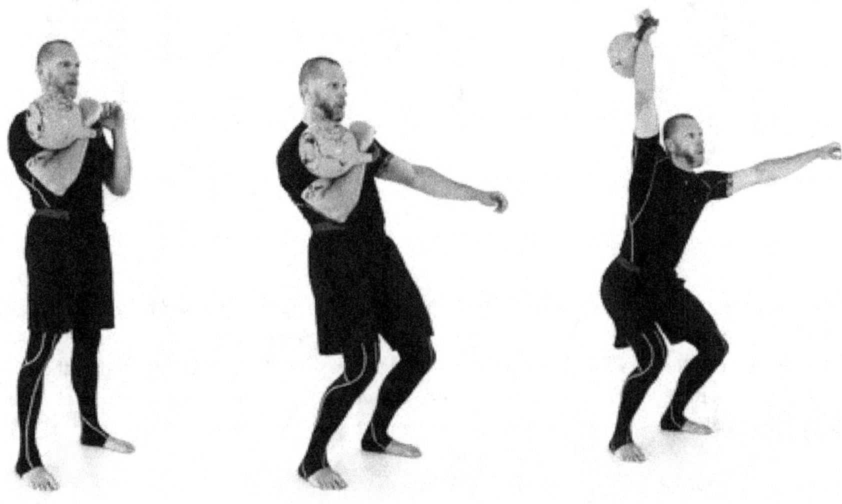

Key safety point to consider. When you're in the under squat you should pay great attention to the alignment of your pelvis. The pelvis should be aligned with your spine, you control this alignment with your gluteus maximus, i.e. through contraction which pulls the pelvis back in line with the spine.

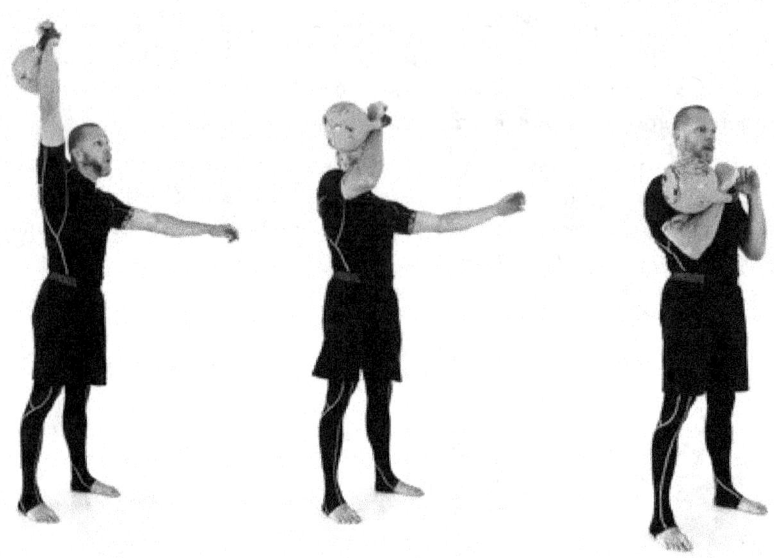

The easiest way to think about the jerk is to push your knees forward and back immediately, this is to push the weight up, then you drop your hips low to come under the weight and push yourself away from the weight. There is no pressing in the jerk. Once you're under the weight and everything is solid and not moving you come up out of the under squat after which you keep the weight overhead for a split second without movement.

The jerk is often combined with the clean, i.e. clean and jerk, and this combo is also used in Kettlebell Sport, which is like the CrossFit Games or Olympics for kettlebells.

Bonus videos:
Kettlebell Jerk In Slow-mo go.cavemantraining.com/kbe-vid-90
Difference Between Clean And Press/Push Press/Jerk go.cavemantraining.com/kbe-vid-91
Kettlebell Clean And Jerk Different Angles In Slow-mo go.cavemantraining.com/kbe-vid-92

Bonus workouts:
Prometheus go.cavemantraining.com/kbe-vid-93
Clean and jerk marathon go.cavemantraining.com/kbe-vid-94

An interesting read: Kettlebell Sport—The Martial Art for Survivors, Pacifists, and Peacemakers go.cavemantraining.com/kbe-vid-95

Rear Press

There is the front, side, and then there is the rear press. You won't hear much about it as it's an unconventional press I started using when I wrote *Master The Kettlebell Press*. It's a press variation that has to be approached with care, not because the exercise is dangerous, but because the progression is one that requires time due to humans never pressing from this angle.

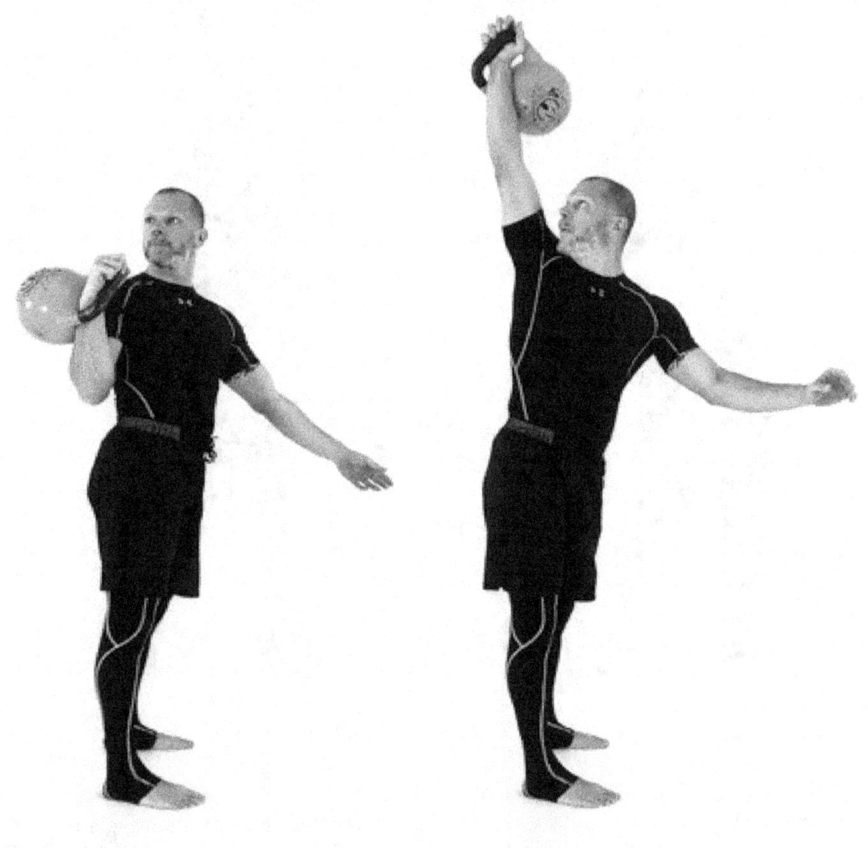

Before you can rear press you need good thoracic rotation, if you lack the ability to create good solid rotation through the thoracic spine then the rear press is not an exercise you should attempt. This variation of the press is not to be confused with the spiral or rotational press, those two are where you come in and out of thoracic rotation, with this variation you stay in thoracic rotation and press at the rear.

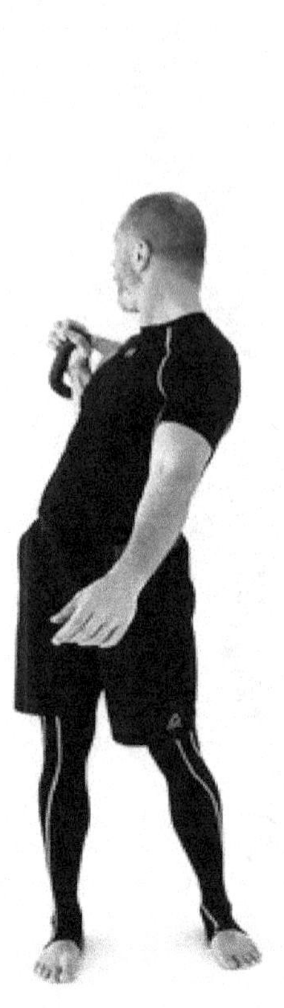 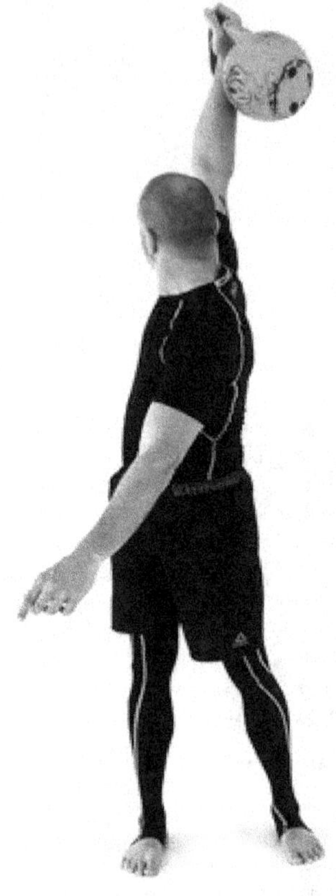

Your starting position for this press is with thoracic rotation, this means that the angle is created with the spine rather than the hips. Once the rotation is created and the elbow is at the back then the press is initiated, during the press, the objective is to keep moving toward medial and up. This exercise hits the rear deltoids.

I must double stress that the exercise is one that requires long progression starting with lightweight.

Seated Press

The seated press adds complexity (good) to the press exercise by requiring a lot of hip flexion, hence, you need good hamstring flexibility, and you'll also be working your back a whole lot more. You'll see how an easy weight for to press will pretty quickly become much harder to press.

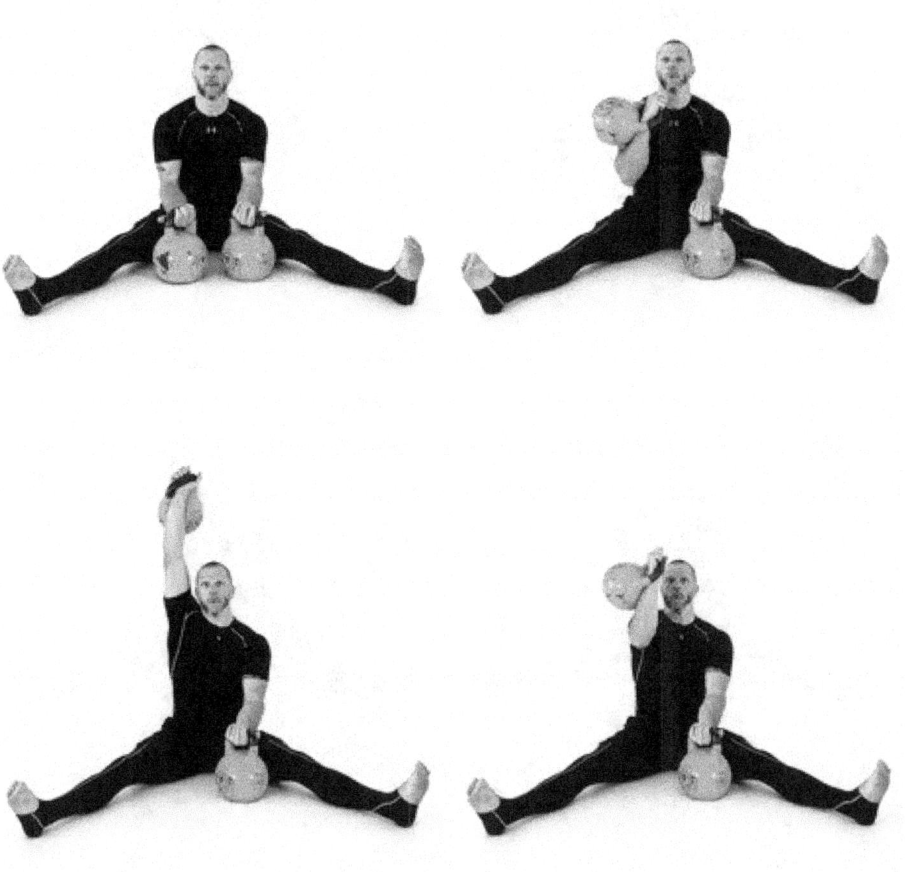

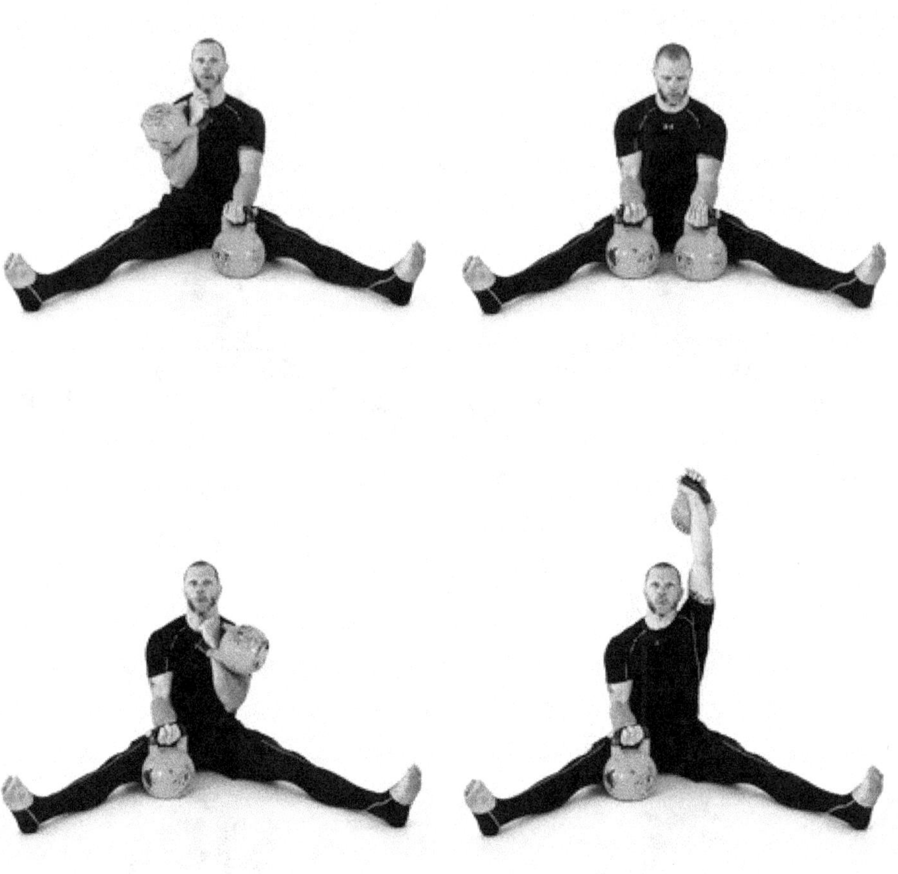

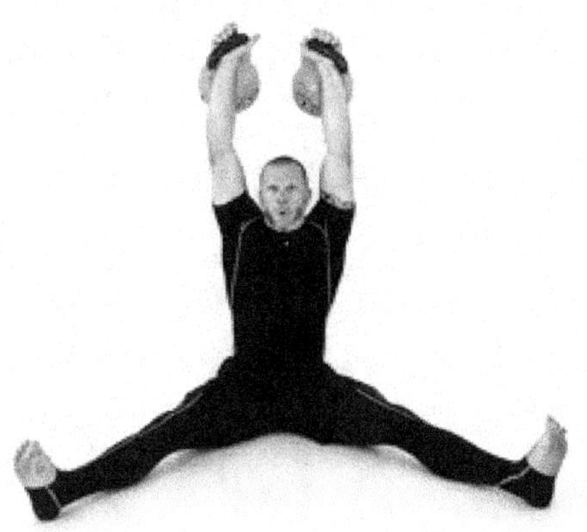

Seated Alternating Press

The benefits of this exercise are hip flexibility, hip and back strength, and of course shoulder strength. Use the curl to reset and pull your pelvis forward upon each alternating rep, don't stay in the same position which will deteriorate over reps, reset, and improve your position. You're not only working flexibility in flexion but also in hip abduction (working your hip abductors and stretching your adductors).

- Sit down
- Spread the legs as wide as possible
- Push the knees into the ground
- Keep pulling the legs out
- Push your buttocks into the ground
- Brace the core
- Pull the top of the pelvis forward and feel the stretch in the gluteals
- Curl the weight
- Rack
- Push the chest out (work the back)
- Press up overhead
- Try and stay overhead for a second or so
- Lower into rack
- Lower to the ground

- Alternate sides

Bonus workouts:
- Kettlebell Workout NEMESIS go.cavemantraining.com/kbe-vid-96

Seesaw Press

The difference between a seesaw press and alternating press is that with the seesaw press both kettlebells keep moving and with the alternating press one waits for the other before moving. Either of these presses is always performed with two weights.

The seesaw press is great for the thoracic area and it's also a real shoulder burner because the tension remains on the deltoids throughout the exercise. The tension remains because of the movement not returning to racking (chest/rest). Your objective is to mimic a real seesaw which is one side up while the other goes down with constant movement.

The alternating press has one weight waiting in recking position for the other to return and then go up. The alternating press can also be performed with a front or side press, whereas the seesaw press is always performed with a side press.

The seesaw press should be programmed in lower reps than the alternating press due to the constant pressure on the deltoids. A lower weight is also recommended. The opposing shoulders/shoulder blades moving is what provides the benefits for the thoracic area, it's not just the movement but also the stabilization requirements throughout the movement that is great from this exercise.

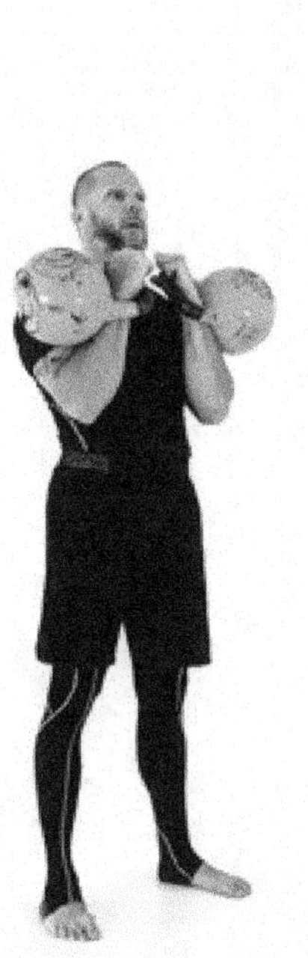
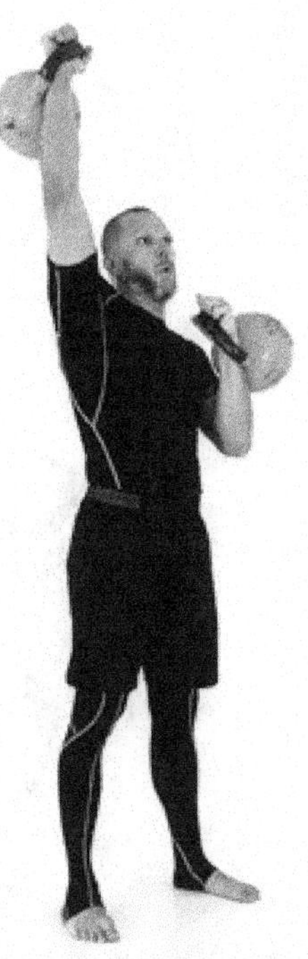

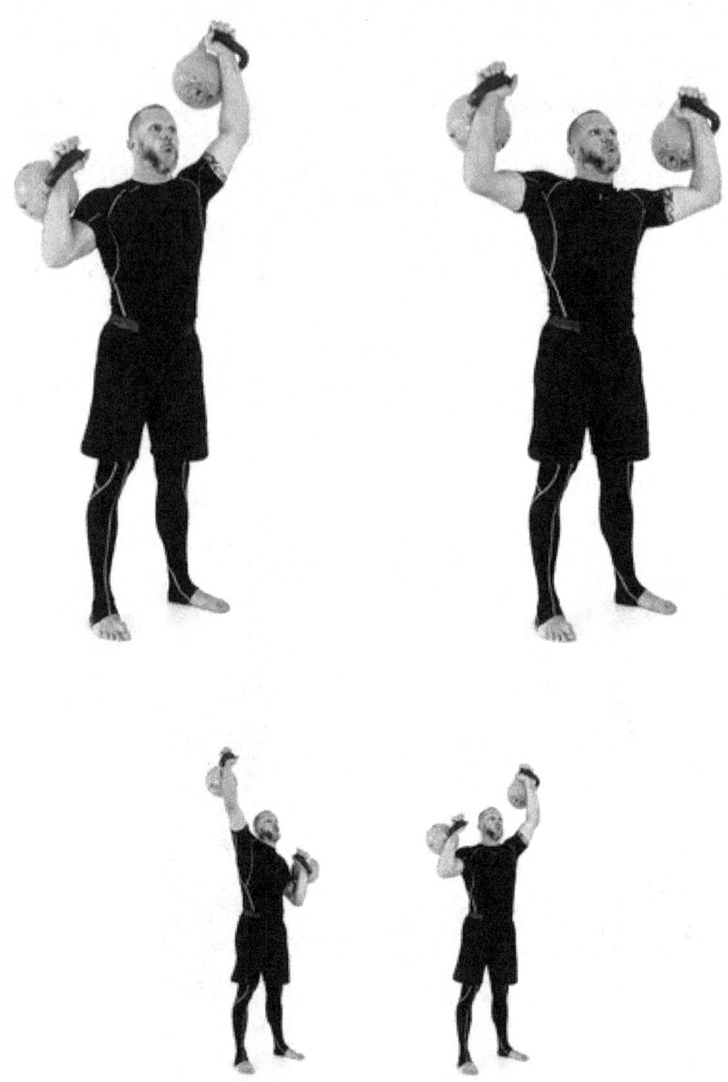

Bonus workouts:
- The Man Of Steel Workout go.cavemantraining.com/kbe-vid-97

Side Press

The side press is a great variation to target the lateral part of the deltoid. Bringing the kettlebell out to the side really challenges your stabilizers and you'll feel your obliques and quadratus lumborum having to do a whole lot more work. Put the feet closer together, grab two kettlebells to side press on both sides at the same time and you have the military press.

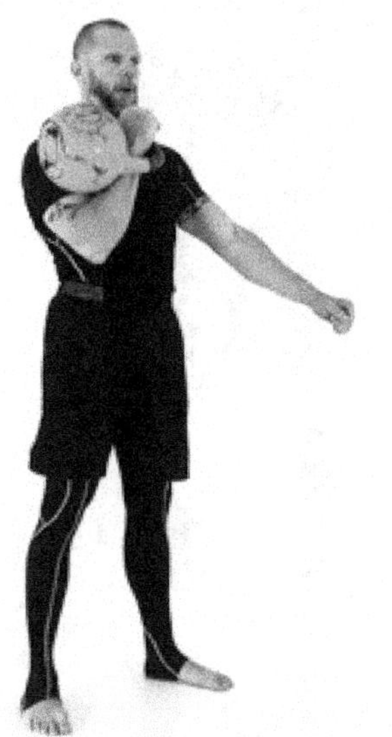 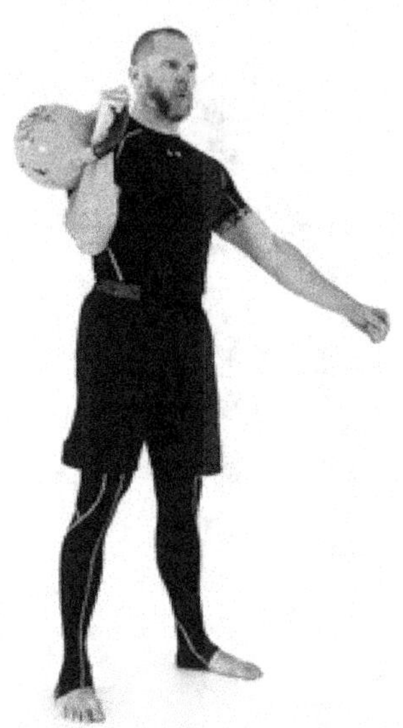

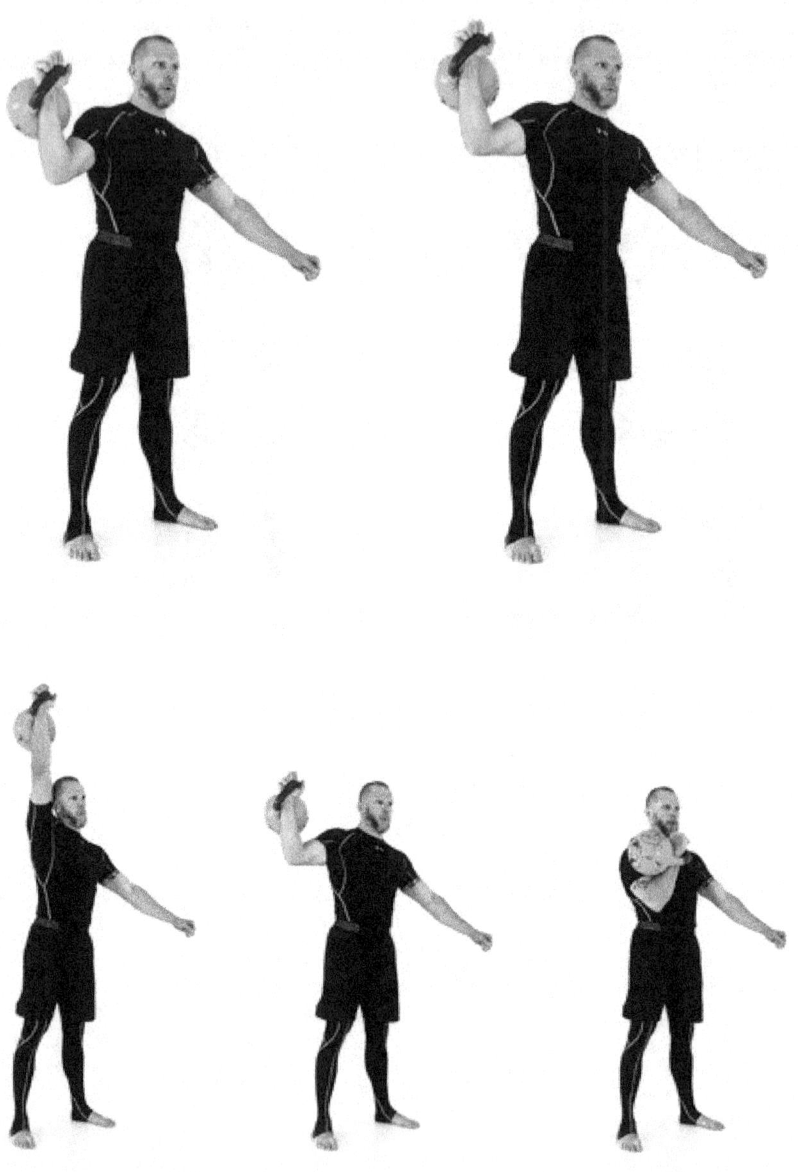

The side press' trajectory is half a circle out to the side.

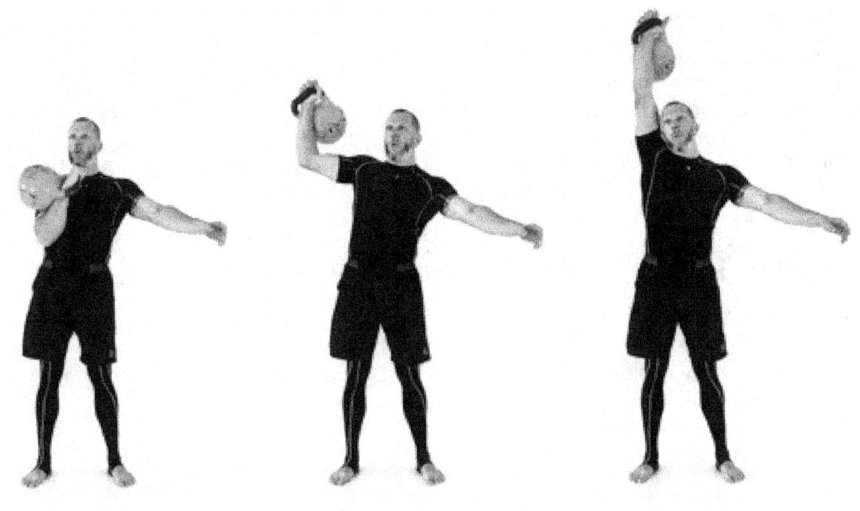

Bonus videos:
The Difference Between Front And Side Shoulder Press go.cavemantraining.com/kbe-vid-98
Military Press VS Overhead Press go.cavemantraining.com/kbe-vid-99

Bonus workouts:
Iron Man Workout go.cavemantraining.com/kbe-vid-100

Sots Press

The Sots press is an incredibly advanced exercise with lots of benefits, hence, an exercise you should include in your training. To be able to perform a good Sots press takes time and you'll need to master the squat first, then back strength, followed by a good overhead position, and finally add load and press from the bottom of the squat. This is more a back workout than it is a shoulder workout and if you can press a 40kg weight you'll be humbled by the Sots press and find out that you'll have to start at ¼ of your weight to progress.

This kettlebell exercise is great for so many things, but here are a few to mention:

- ➢ Shoulder stability
- ➢ Range of motion
- ➢ Working on creating and maintaining tension throughout the body
- ➢ Squat depth
- ➢ Stability

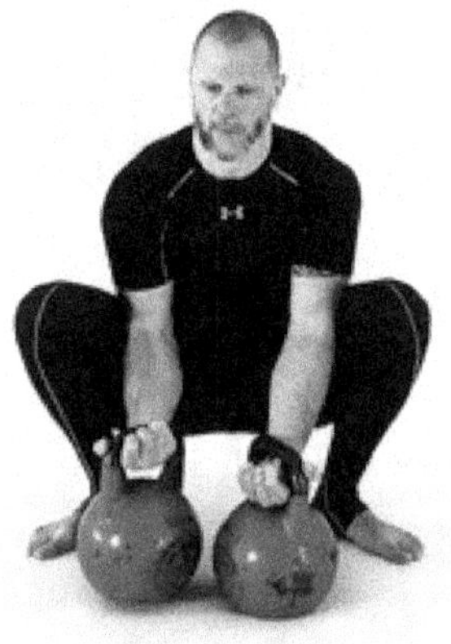
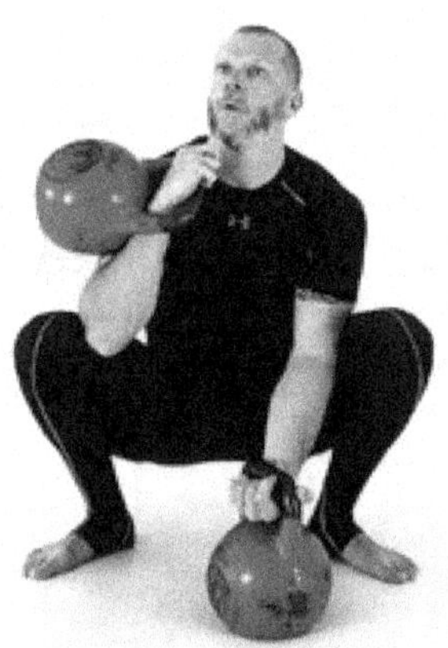

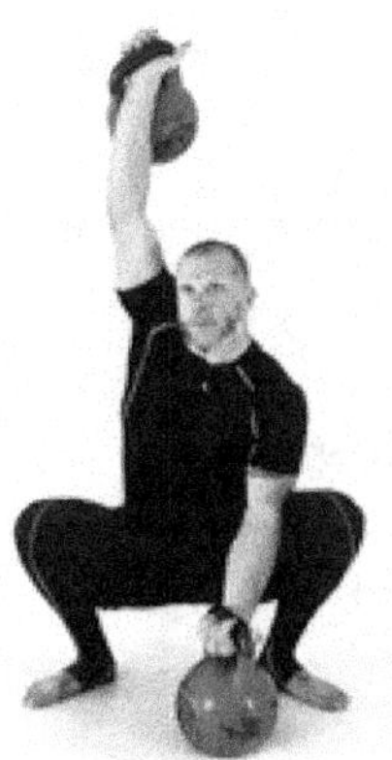 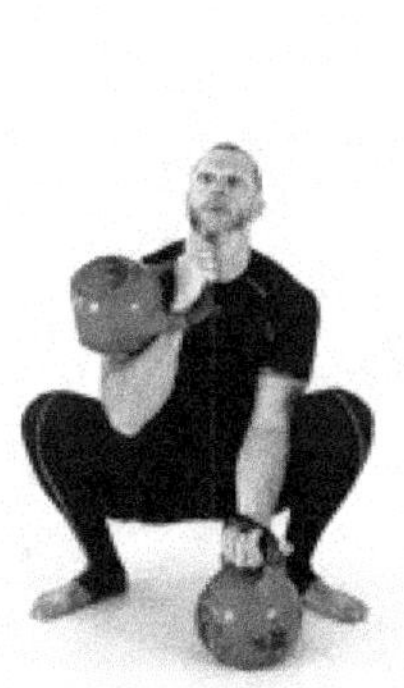 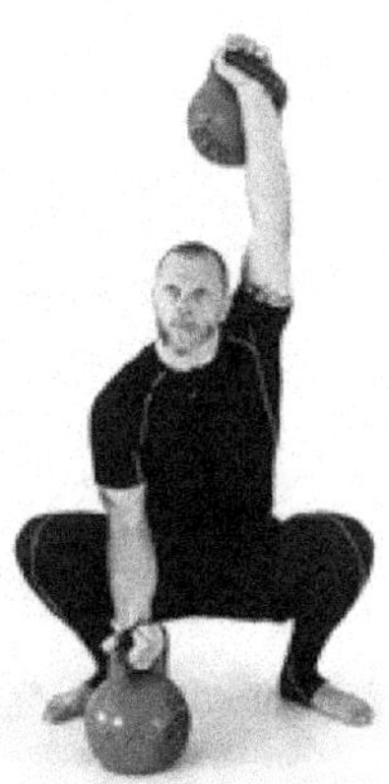

Working with one kettlebell on the ground can help you with balance, you lightly hold on to the kettlebell on the ground and use as an additional counterbalance while pressing overhead. You should use this if you're having trouble falling back. You can also use this to add an additional pull down into the squat and work the elbow flexors, i.e. you lightly curl the weight, but not so much that it leaves the ground. This adds load to the squat but also provides some stability.

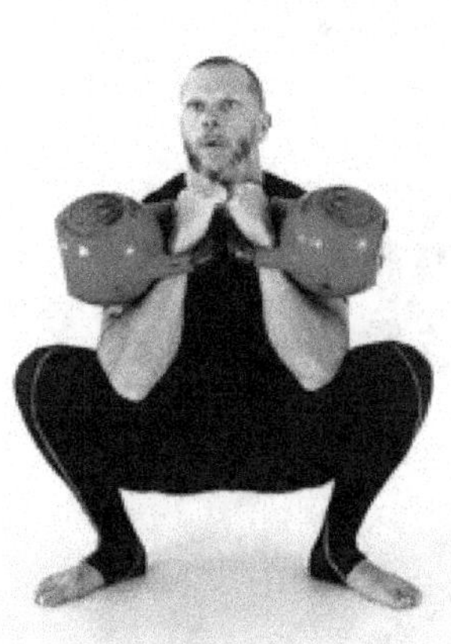 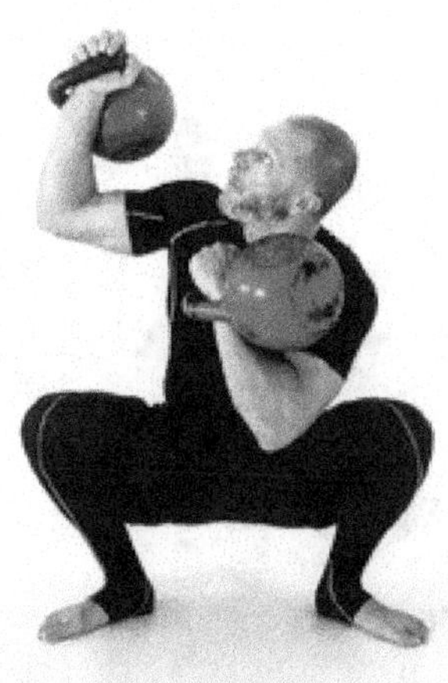

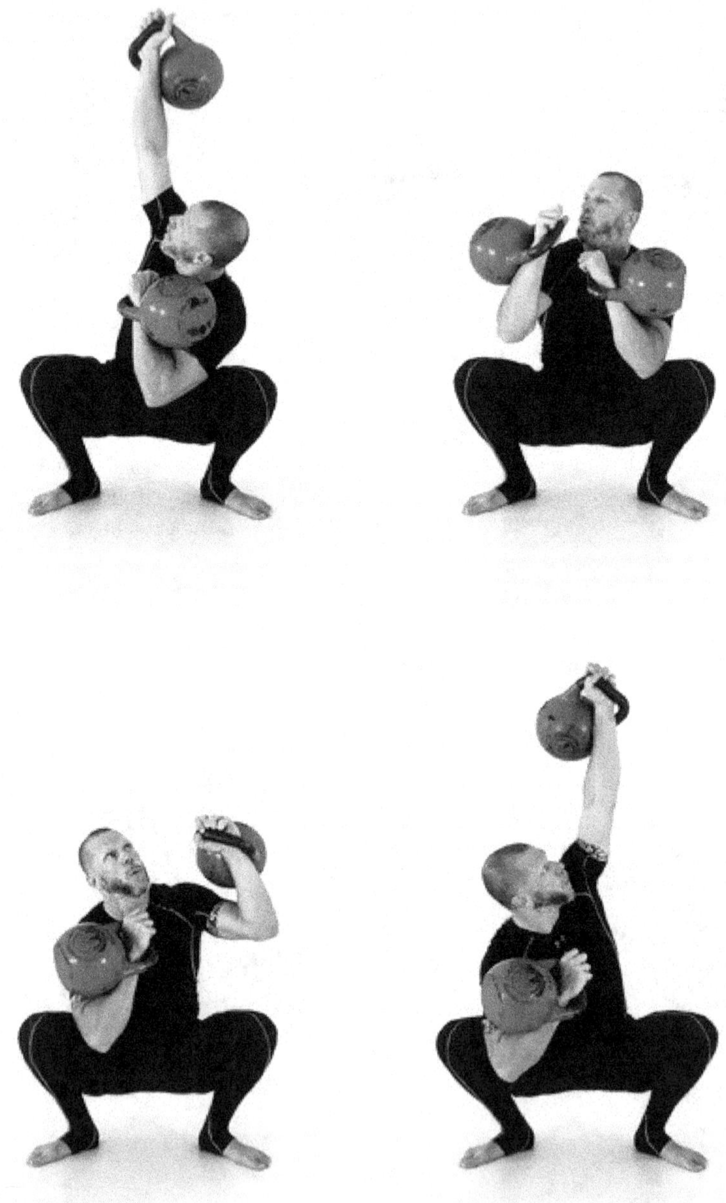

A Sots press can be paired with thoracic rotation during the progression to the full position which is without rotation and looking ahead. In the sequence above thoracic rotation is used to make the press easier, but you should also use this variation to simply work on thoracic rotation.

To perform:

- Come into a deep squat
- Keep tension in the squat
- Don't hunch or sag into the squat
- Press the feet into the ground
- Contract the gluteals for hip stabilization
- Pull the gluteus maximus to pull the pelvis as upright as possible or required
- Stay an inch above your max squat depth
- Contract the erector spinae muscle groups for thoracic hyperextension
- Pack everything around the chest and shoulder blades
- You've now created a stable base to press from

When pressing up straight

- Keep the elbow directly under the weight
- Keep the forearm close to vertical
- Look ahead
- Press up in a direct path to the endpoint
- Start pulling down with the lat as much as required to keep the shoulder safe
- Engage the triceps
- Press till full lockout above the shoulder
- Return to racking in reverse
- Repeat or lower to the ground with an eccentric curl

When pressing with thoracic rotation

- Initiate thoracic rotation
- Initiate the press
- Look at the weight
- Bring the elbow laterally out during the press
- Keep rotating
- Engage the triceps

- Press till full lockout above the shoulder

- Return to racking in reverse

- Repeat or lower to the ground with an eccentric curl

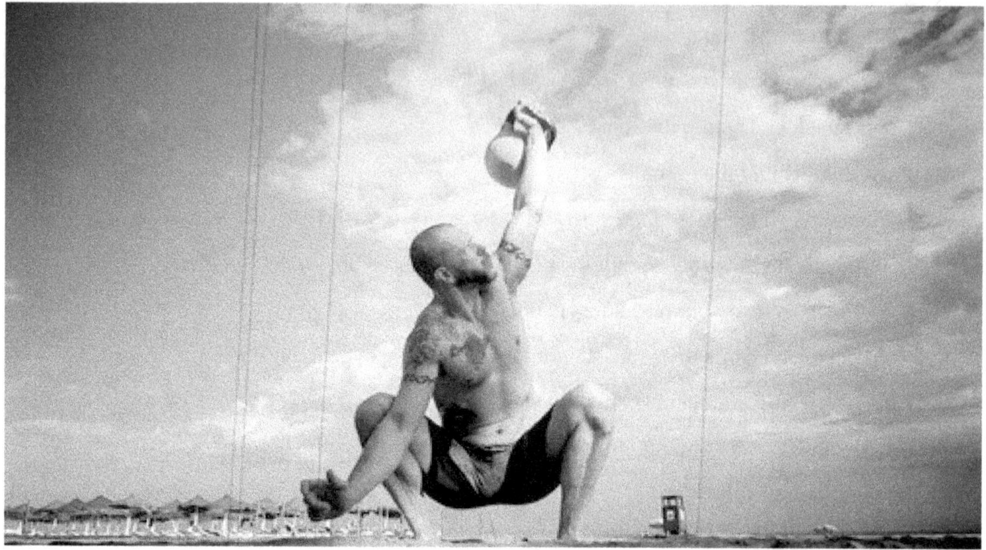

Pressing the non-pressing arm against the knee and out will assist with stabilization.

I very much like the alternating Sots press because it has several exercises into one, squat, curl and press. All of these things require progression, great precision, and flawless technique. Proper hand insertion. Rotating at the right time. Creating tension in the right areas and maintain that. And so on.

If you're performing the Sots press with one kettlebell you can choose to rotate at the thoracic spine, the rotation will make the press easier and there is nothing wrong with using this for progression to the neutrally-aligned Sots press, plus your objective might be to work the thoracic. Thoracic rotation is an area most athletes neglect.

Before you attempt this exercise you will need to be able to squat deep properly, being able to keep the torso upright and heels on the ground.

"One of the most incredible kettlebell exercises you can do for strength, flexibility and mobility in one. Every CrossFit box should incorporate this exercise into their mobility sessions." ~ Taco Fleur

Bonus workouts:
FUSION4.5 Kettlebell Workout go.cavemantraining.com/kbe-vid-102
The Man of Steel Workout go.cavemantraining.com/kbe-vid-103

Spiral Press

The kettlebell spiral press is an exercise I designed to work the thoracic spine. This exercise should be performed with a light to medium weight, but once you're conditioned for this movement it can also be used to create the initial momentum for pressing heavier weights, just like the leg push is used in the push press. You will find a video in your online course.

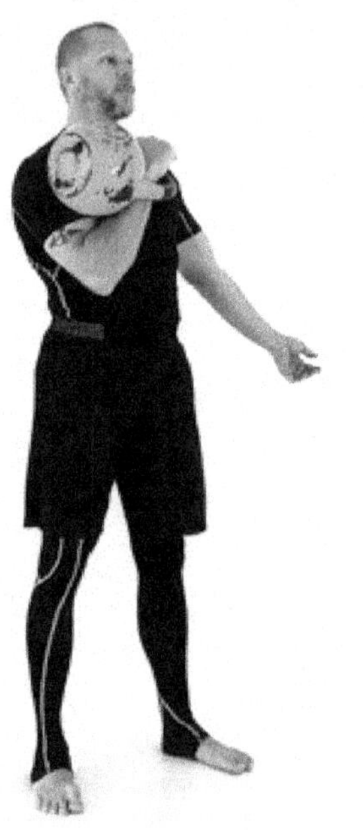 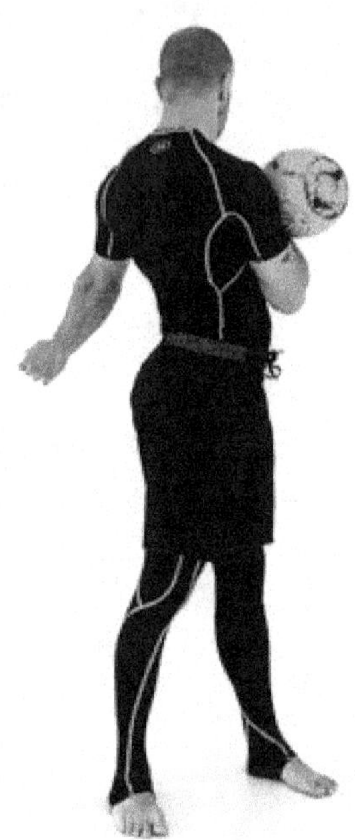

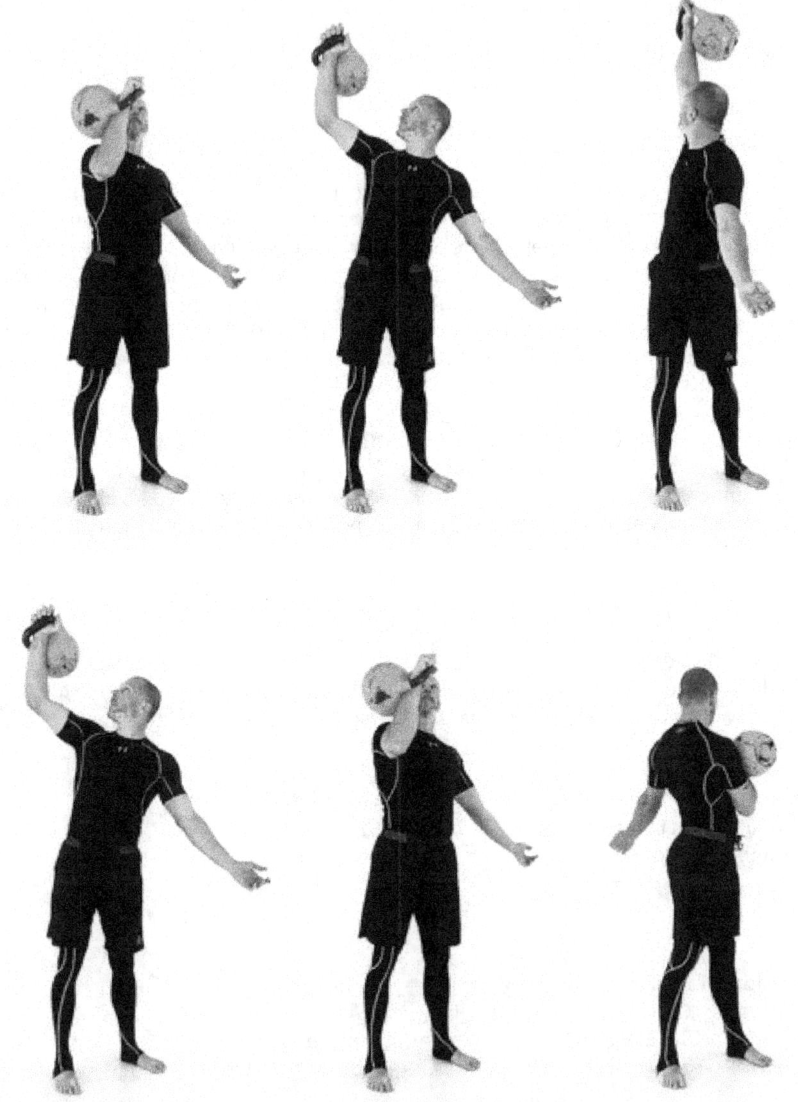

Why:
  • Thoracic spine mobility
  • Shoulder strength
  • Shoulder stability
  • Core stability

- Multifidus
- Rotatores
- Obliques
- Thoracic spine rotation
- Shoulder extension
- Shoulder abduction
- Elbow extension

Rotation in the T-spine is something that does not occur in the day to day lives of many people, especially office workers, hence, this is an area that needs to be approached carefully. The muscles need to be conditioned slowly and step-by-step. Perform bodyweight exercises that involve thoracic spine rotation regularly before attempting the spiral press. If you have good thoracic mobility then this is an easier exercise to work on a good straight overhead press, i.e. better shoulder mobility. The straight overhead press would require more shoulder mobility than the spiral press, hence, this is a great exercise to use for progression to the overhead press, assuming the person in question has good thoracic mobility.

It should be noted that the one might create lateral thoracic flexion during the rotation when the shoulder mobility is lacking. It's not recommended for beginners to create both lateral flexion and rotation of the spine at the same time but instead focus on one pattern separately. Once advanced and done with intention, not to gain range, then this is perfectly fine under light load and controlled movement.

To perform:
1. Neutral stance
2. Kettlebell racked on one side
3. Hold the non-working arm out to the side with slight tension from the fist to shoulder
4. Rotate into the non-working arm through contraction and not through swinging
5. Rotate into the opposite side
6. Press up as the kettlebell moves through a spiral pattern
7. Eyes on the bell from the moment it reaches eye level
8. Return the bell via the same path
9. Repeat the pattern

Bonus videos:
Kettlebell Rotational Exercises For The Core go.cavemantraining.com/kbe-vid-104
2 Kettlebell Mobility Combos go.cavemantraining.com/kbe-vid-105
10 KB Exercises To Challenge ROM go.cavemantraining.com/kbe-vid-106
CAVEMANROM—Kettlebells For Flexibility And Mobility go.cavemantraining.com/kbe-vid-107

Bonus workouts:
Kronos go.cavemantraining.com/kbe-vid-108

Kettlebell Push-up

Similar to the press, you exert physical force on the kettlebell, but in this case, it's in order to move yourself away from it. A push-up done on the floor would be pushing yourself away from the floor. If you take the same push-up position and turn it around—laying flat—and perform the same movement it becomes as press as you're moving the object away from yourself.

Using a kettlebell for push-ups may seem redundant, and if you're just doing normal push-ups it probably is, unless it just becomes easier to do the push-ups off the kettlebells so that it all flows. The part where the kettlebell becomes interesting to use for push-ups is where the kettlebell provides instability and/or elevation.

Bottoms-up Push-up

The bottoms-up push-up can be done with one or two kettlebells. The kettlebells are placed upside down with the base facing up and the athlete balancing with the hands placed on the base during the push-up. More details coming in the updated version of the encyclopedia. See the introduction on how to get your updated version.

Bonus videos:
Bottoms-up Push-up go.cavemantraining.com/kbe-vid-142

Archer Push-up

The archer push-up is where the kettlebell is used as an elevation and the extended arm rests on the bell while the other arm is used to push up. More details coming in the updated version of the encyclopedia. See the introduction on how to get your updated version.

Bonus videos:
The Dudley Workout With Archer Push-up go.cavemantraining.com/kbe-vid-143

Crush Grip Push-up

This variation of the push-up is where the athlete balances on the bell through a crush grip, meaning, if the athlete would not crush the bell he/she would slip off it. More details coming in the updated version of the encyclopedia. See the introduction on how to get your updated version.

Bonus videos:
Crush Grip Push-up go.cavemantraining.com/kbe-vid-144

Triceps Push-up

The triceps push-up is where the bells are placed right under the shoulders and the athlete performs a triceps push-up while gripping the handles. More details coming in the updated version of the encyclopedia. See the introduction on how to get your updated version.

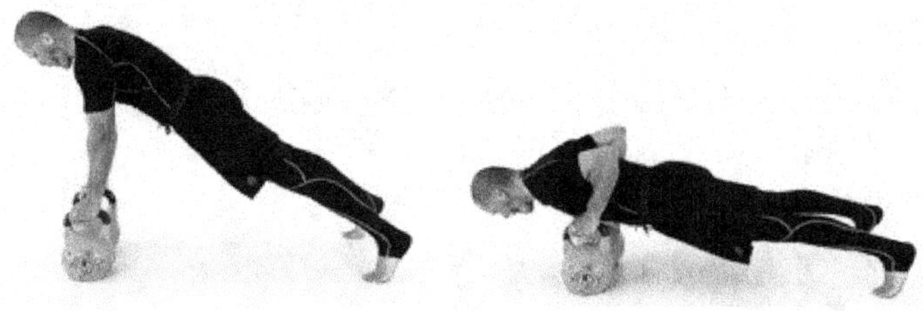

Bonus videos:
How To Use Triceps Push-up In A Combo go.cavemantraining.com/kbe-vid-145

Kettlebell Row

Kettlebell rows are a great exercise to work the back and can be performed from dead or hang position. The dead row is great for heavier lower reps due to the weight returning dead to the ground each time and releasing tension. The hang row is great for keeping tension and faster reps with lighter weight.

The kettlebell row variations with the static hip hinge (bent-over) are also a great gluteal and back exercise due to the isometric hold required (erector spinae and gluteals). You can remove the work needed to be done by the back through changing the stance, the least amount of work required by the back will be when using one weight and one hand/elbow/arm on the knee.

Kettlebell rows are great to work the rear deltoids when you keep the elbows tucked in nicely and row into the hips removing work done by the biceps.

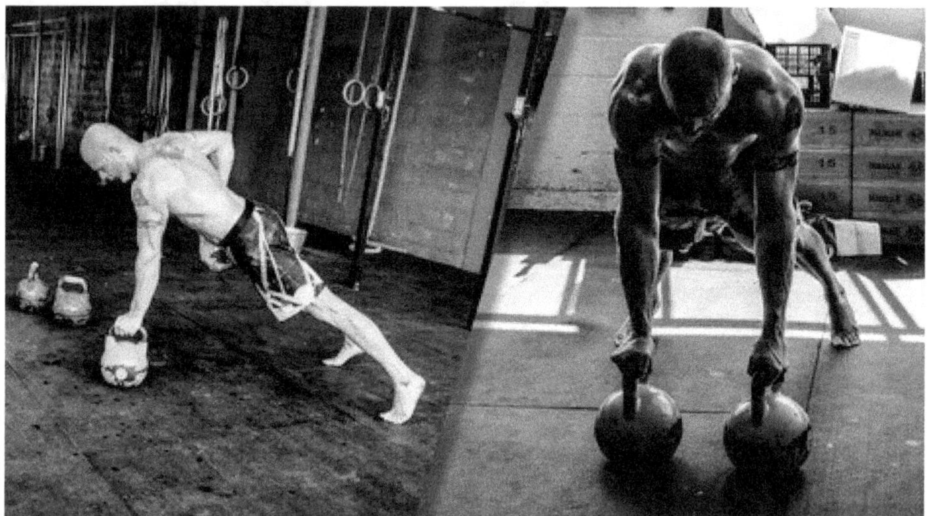

Dot points:
- You can row while supporting the torso or without
- Rowing without support challenges the core muscles more
- Rowing with support allows you to isolate and focus on the row more
- Relax the elbow flexors while rowing
- Pull the elbow back into the hip and past
- If the weight starts dead on the ground it's a dead row
- If your hand is coming toward the shoulder then you're curling instead of rowing
- Control the movement and get from it why you're working out for
- Master the movement first and then go high reps and heavier weight
- Nothing but the arms that are working should be moving
- The bigger the angle between the elbow and ribs the more emphasis will be placed in the middle of the back
- The closer your elbow is to the body the safer it is for beginners
- There are many more ways to perform the kettlebell row

Renegade Rows

Renegade rows are great for the core, rear deltoids, latissimus dorsi, hips, and even quads.

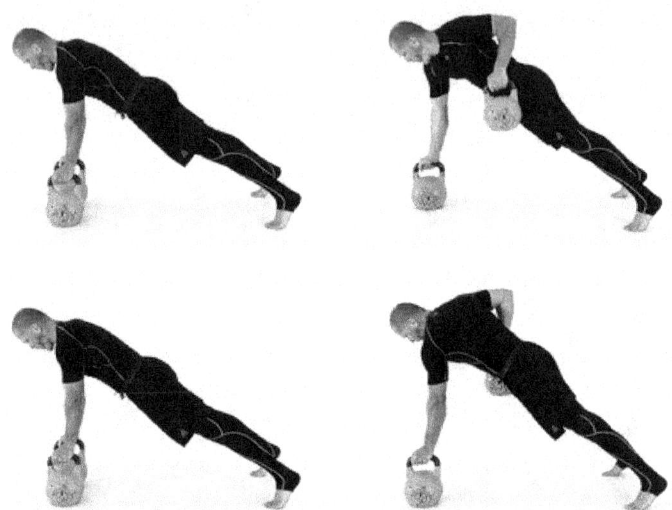

The most popular variation of this involves a push-up. A triceps push-up to be exact, due to where the kettlebells are placed—under the shoulders—you can't perform a chest push-up.

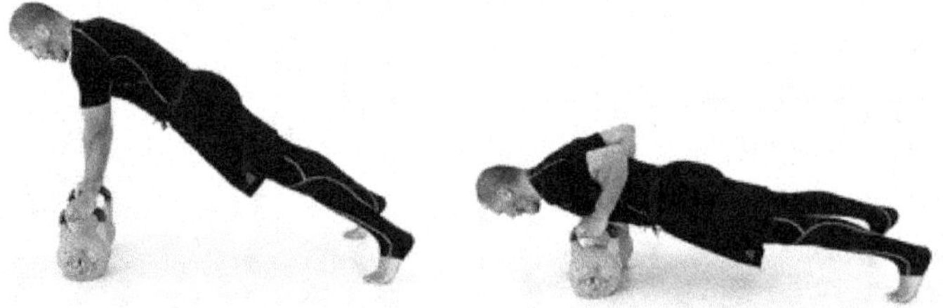

To get in position:
* Stand with the feet outside of the kettlebells

- Come down into a squat
- Lock the elbows
- Brace the chest
- Kick the legs out

To perform:

- Plank position
- Lats active throughout to protect the shoulders
- Everything is tight
- Row one kettlebell
  - Shoulder braced
  - Chest braced
  - Tight abs
  - Hips locked
  - Knees locked
  - Row toward the hip
  - Focus on the rear delt doing the work
  - Gently lower the weight back into starting position
  - Starting position is right under the shoulder
- Repeat with the other arm

To come out:

- Prepare to take your weight on the arms
- Kick your legs in
- Feet next to the kettlebells

You only want to do this exercise if you can keep a straight line (ankles, knees, hips, shoulders) throughout the row. If your hips come up into the air then you're better off going with a lighter weight or working on core/hip strength. The alternative is to come into a plank and simply take one hand (support) off the floor for 2 to 3 seconds and then do the other side.

Bonus workouts:
Gorilla Silverback go.cavemantraining.com/kbe-vid-109
Gorilla Blackback go.cavemantraining.com/kbe-vid-110
The Dudley go.cavemantraining.com/kbe-vid-111

Bent-over Rows

A bent-over row position is simply a position in which you're bent-over, it does not dictate the type of row you're performing, i.e. what range (dead or hang), nor the angle. The bent-over rows are performed as per the following photos.

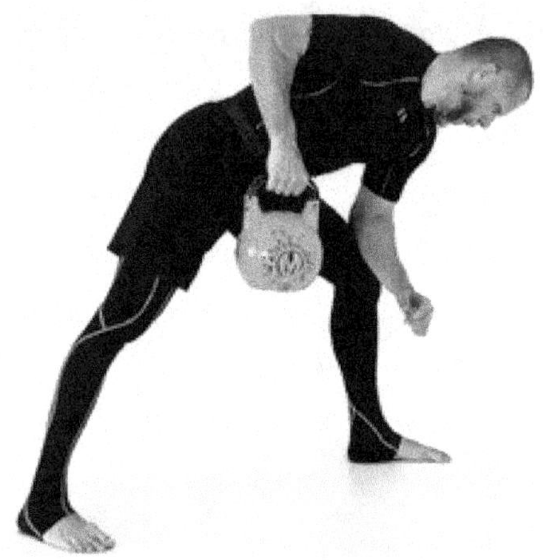

You can perform them as shown in the next sequence which allows you to put your weight on the kettlebell through the non-working arm.

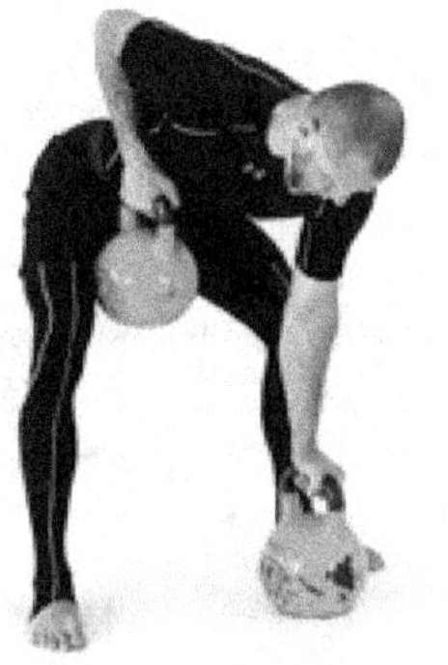 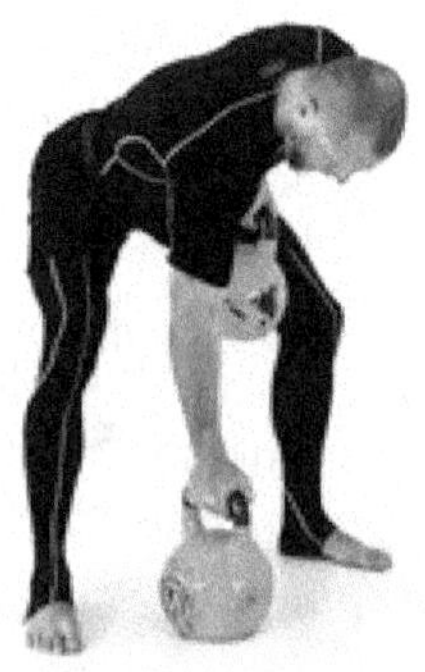

If it feel better, you can also put your feet closer together and row on the outside of the legs as demonstrated in the following sequence of photos.

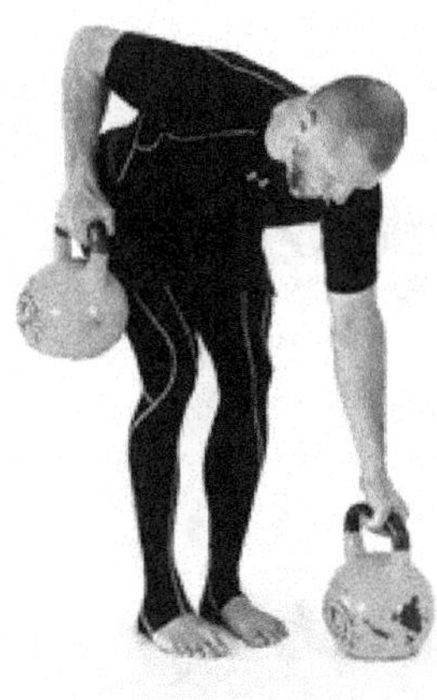 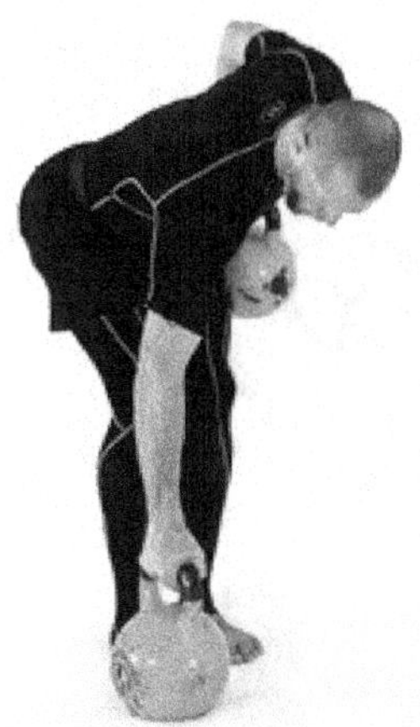

Rows performed with the feet closer together will provider more instability and requires more stabilization. Increased stability allows you to focus on the row and row more weight. Either variation has its advantages as training instability creates stability.

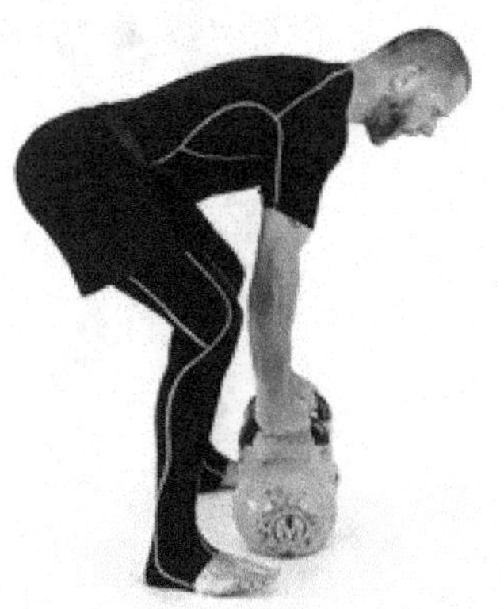 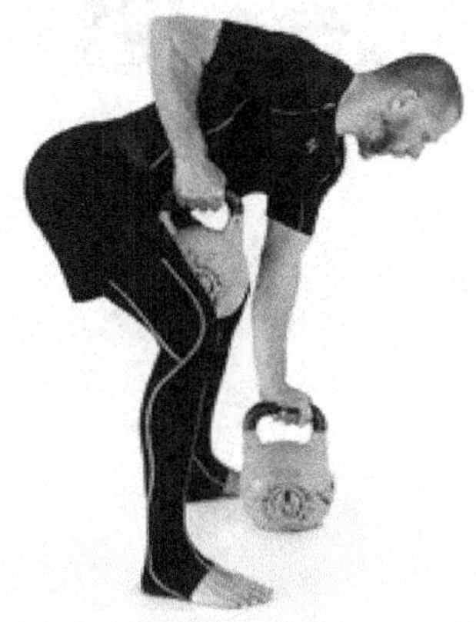

The variation demonstrated above provides the most stability, three points of support, the legs and one arm. This variation would allow you to row the heaviest weight with the best form and technique.

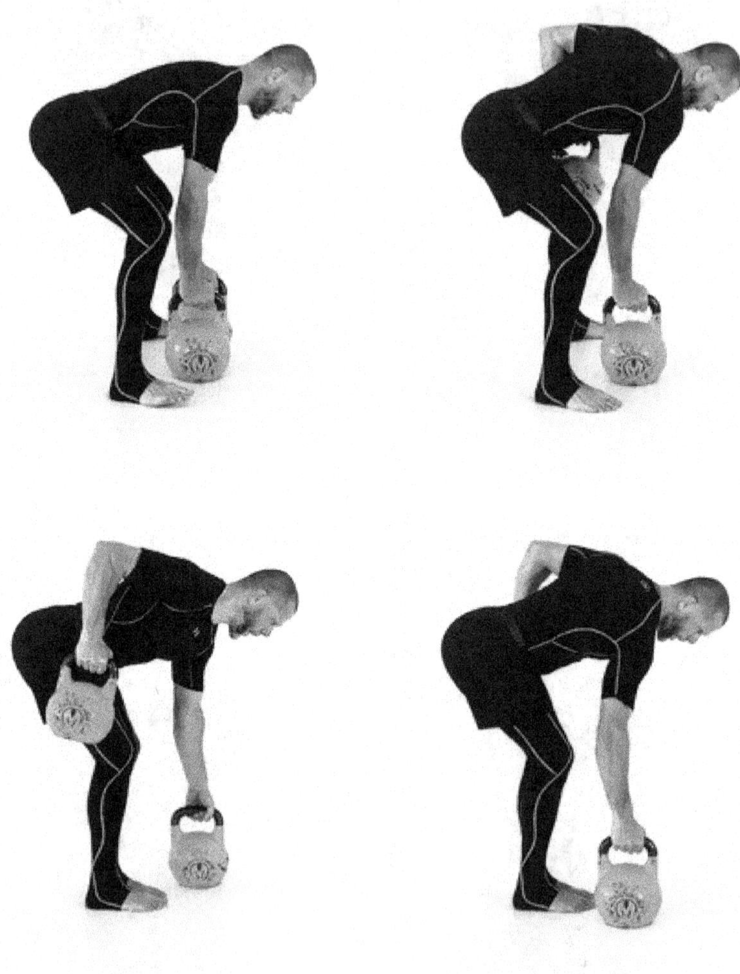

The above two photos demonstrate the feet together and rowing on the outside of the legs, this creates instability and requires good core activation. Taking out the support from the arm would add even more instability, hence, more core work.

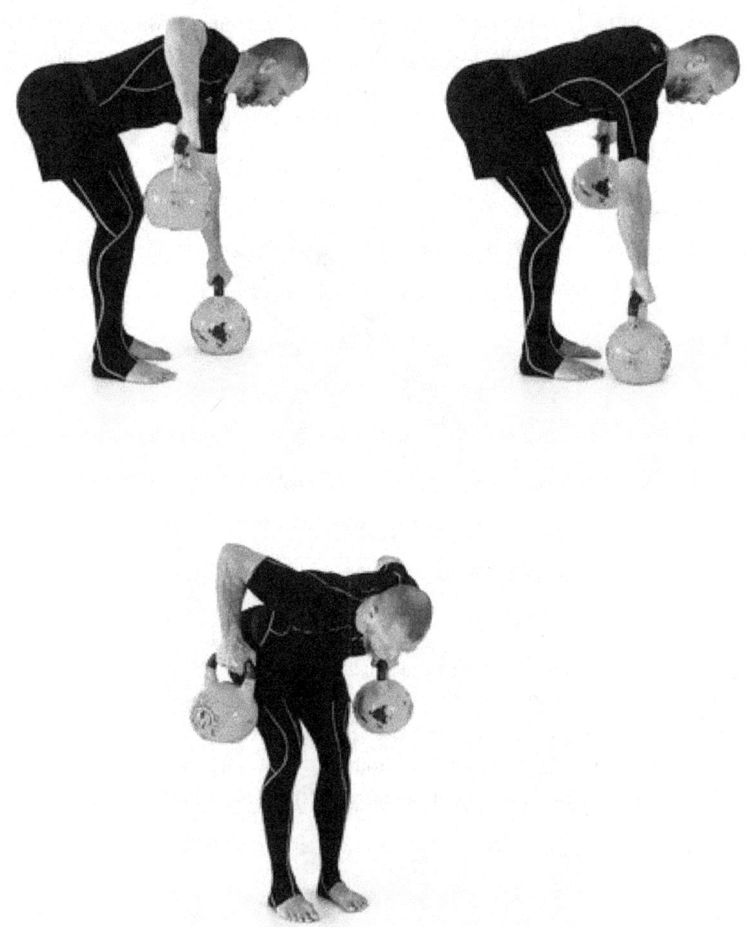

In the last photo the feet are still close together but two kettlebells are rowed at the same time which makes it easier on the core as less stabilization is required due to working with two weights.

Bent-over Dead Rows

All photos have shown the dead row as the weight starts dead, but it can also start in the hand and return to the hang, which means tension remains throughout the reps. The focus of the bent-over row is the rear delt, latissimus dorsi, teres major, and triceps brachii (long head), but there is way more going on as you create a stable base to row/pull the heavyweight from.

A supporting single-arm row position would be when you lunge forward and take a step back to create the position to row from. Your back remains neutral and your non-working arm is resting on the forward knee. Make sure you row and aren't performing bicep curls. If you find that the weight is not moving back and up but remains under and toward the shoulder then you're bicep curling.

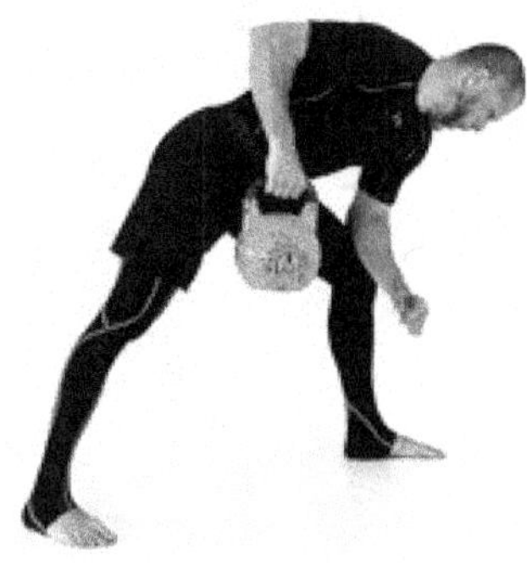

Key safety point to consider. When you first start rowing there is a progression of flexibility that needs to be followed. Your shoulder extension does not have to be exaggerated, it's quite common for people to really want to pull that weight high as the range doesn't feel like a lot. Slowly progress, yes, the higher you come the more range you get but it should not be at the expense of injury. If you have limited range then holding and pausing at a safe range will also get you that time under tension.

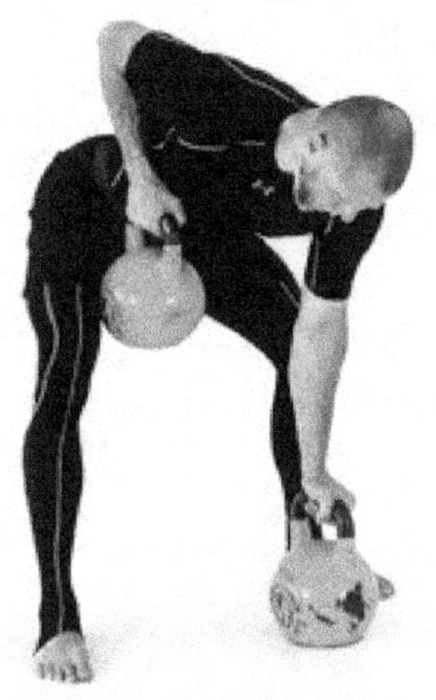 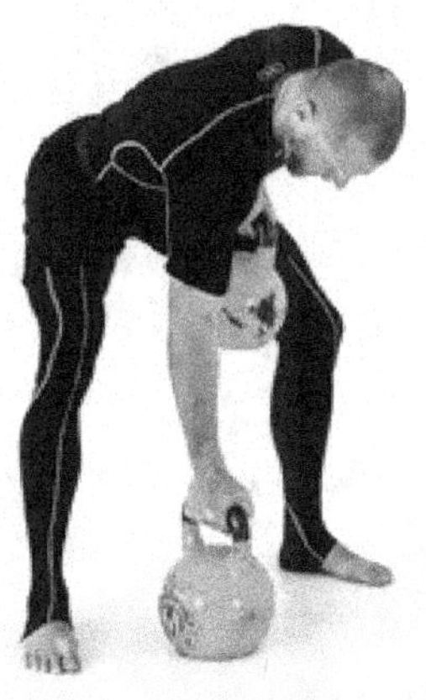

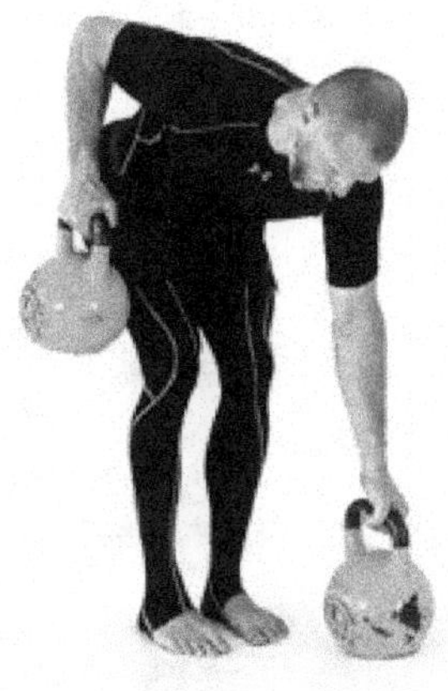 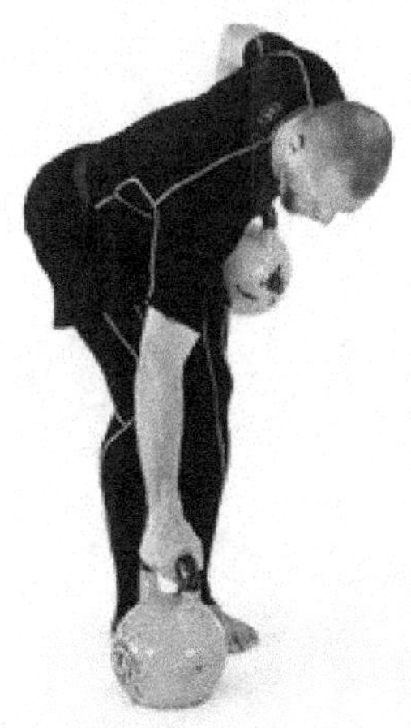

Bonus videos:
Bent-over Dead Row Versus Hang Row go.cavemantraining.com/kbe-vid-112
NR. 1 Mistake Made With Bent-over Rows go.cavemantraining.com/kbe-vid-113
10+ Kettlebell Row Variations go.cavemantraining.com/kbe-vid-114

Bonus workouts:
Prometheus Kettlebell Strength Program go.cavemantraining.com/kbe-vid-115
THE BIG FOUR: Kettlebell Strength Workout go.cavemantraining.com/kbe-vid-116

Kettlebell Snatch

The snatch is a full-body exercise that delivers amazing effects. The snatch can be used to increase cardiovascular endurance, muscular endurance, strength, flexibility, core stability, explosive power, and much more.

The snatch truly works each and every major joint in the body, ankles, knees, hips, shoulders, elbow, and wrists. For strength, you can't deny the major areas that will improve, such as, latissimus dorsi, deltoid, triceps, erector spinae, abdominals, glute, hamstrings, calves, hip flexors, quadriceps, lumbrical muscles, and many more.

All these properties make it the king of kettlebell exercises, an exercise everyone should include in their training.

The snatch is an exercise in which a weight is lifted in one continuous motion from start to overhead with an explosive movement in which the weight arrives at the top through acceleration generated from the start till approximately middle of the full movement.

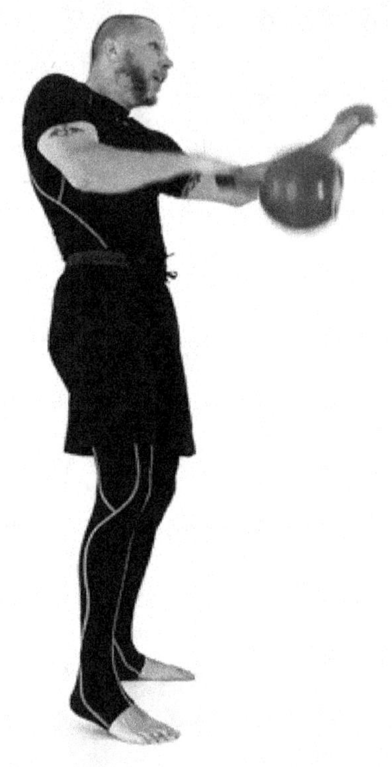

Dead Snatch

The dead snatch is performed with a squat, it can be performed with a hip hinge but is not recommended, not recommended for safety nor for progression. As with any snatch, you can perform a half or a full snatch, the full is from overhead straight to the end (start position) of that variation, whereas the half snatch is from overhead into racking and then to the end of that variation. In the case of a dead snatch full would be from overhead straight to dead, and half would be from overhead to rack and then to dead.

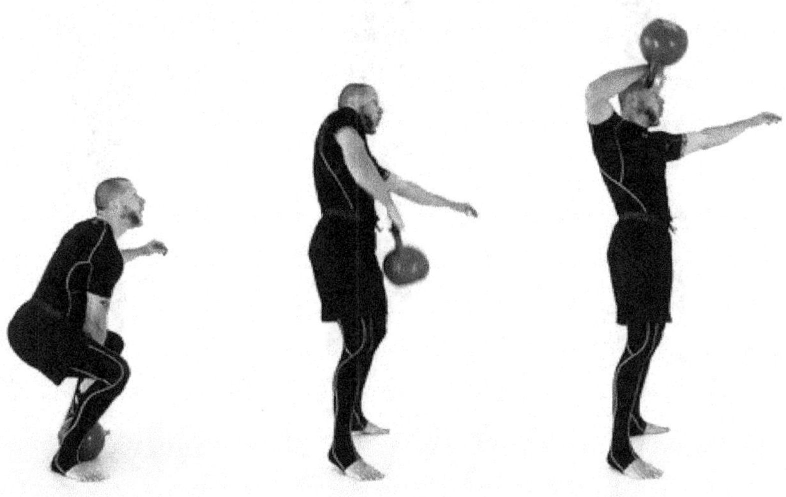

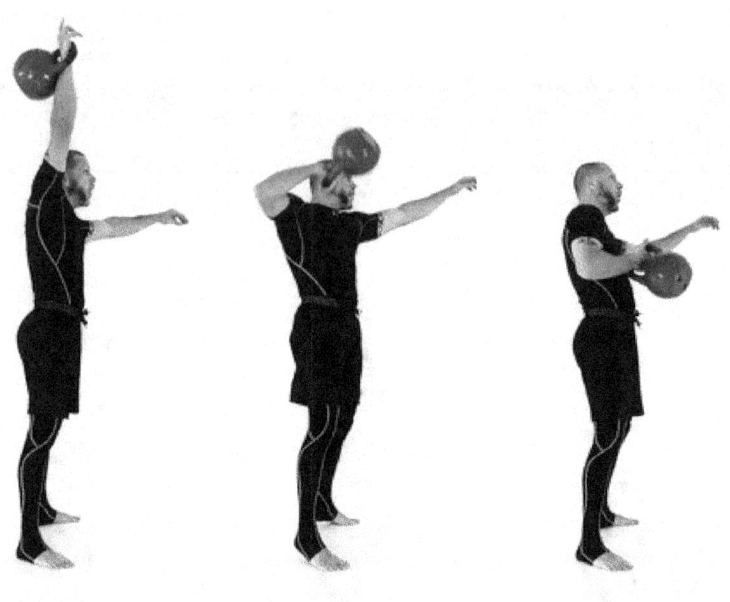

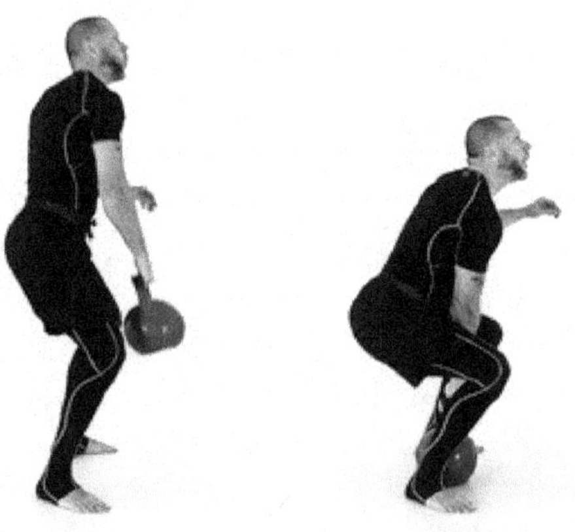

The following sequence demonstrates the half dead snatch. Half means that the weight returns from overhead into racking and then to the ground rather than straight back to the ground.

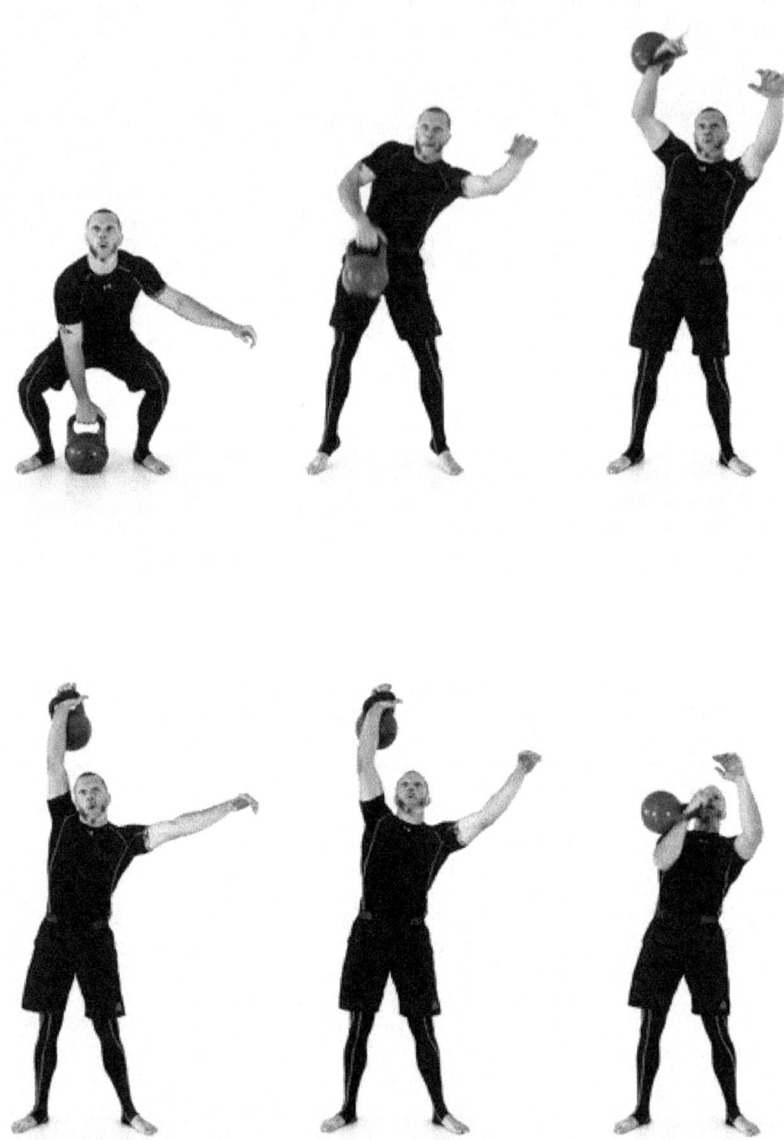

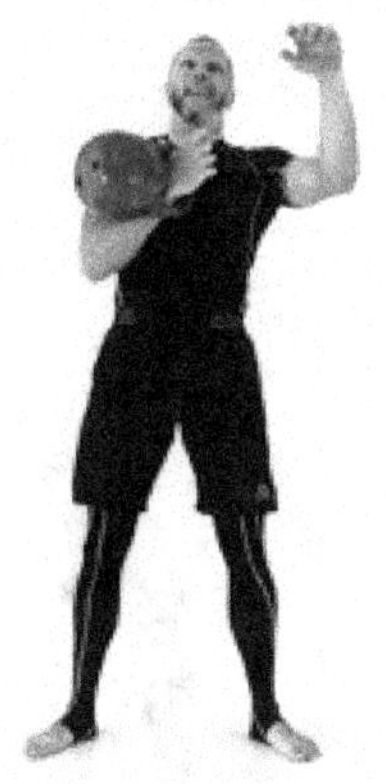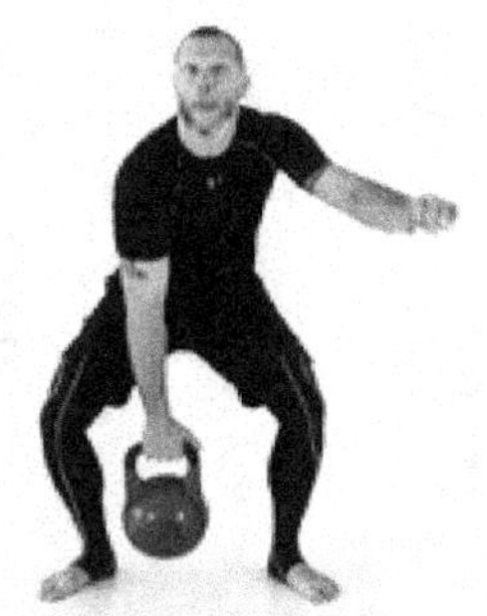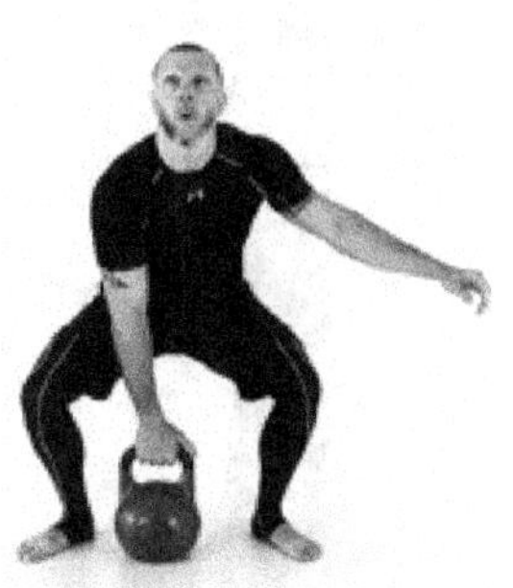

Bonus videos:
The Difference Between A Kettlebell Dead, Swing, And Hang Snatch go.cavemantraining.com/kbe-vid-117
Kettlebell Dead Snatch With Path Of Travel go.cavemantraining.com/kbe-vid-118

Bonus workouts:
CTCF100 Challenge go.cavemantraining.com/kbe-vid-119

Hang Snatch

The hang snatch is almost the same as the dead snatch with the difference being that the kettlebell does not return dead to the ground upon each rep but ends in the hang. The hang snatch is more taxing than the dead snatch because the length for acceleration (pull) and deceleration (drop) is shorter. More power is required for this version of the snatch.

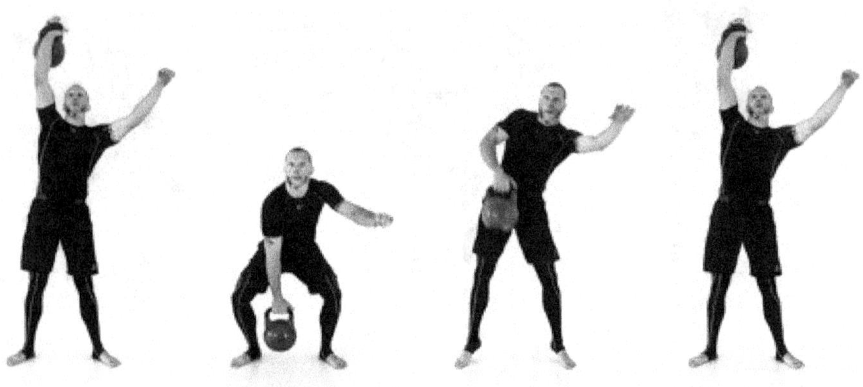

There is no pause in the hang so the exercise becomes a lot more dynamic than the dead snatch where you will at least have a split second of no tension.

Half Snatch

AKA Half swing snatch

The half snatch is where the kettlebell is snatched overhead and then dropped into racking position. This version of the snatch is much easier than the full snatch where the kettlebell goes from overhead into a full drop back into the backswing, hang, or dead to the ground. In the following sequence, the description covers the half snatch with a hip hinge.

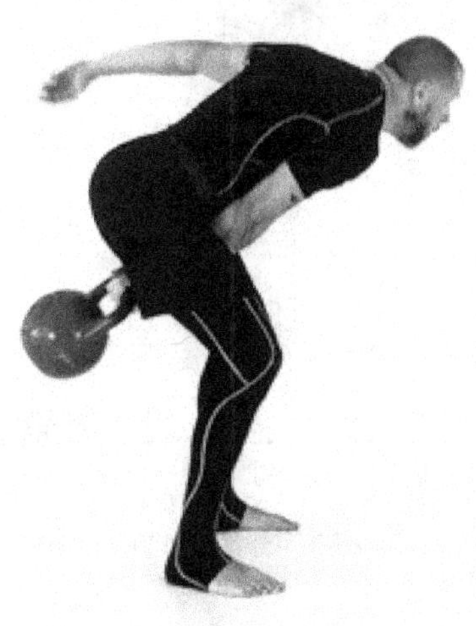

The kettlebell is inserted deep.

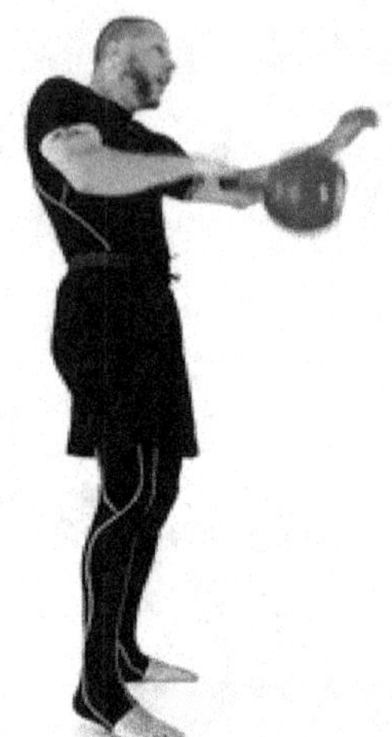

The kettlebell is pulled out and the arm disconnects early. If this was the pendulum swing, the ankles would dorsiflex (knees coming forward) and the hips would follow, keeping the arm connected.

The swing is followed by a shrug pull through hip and thoracic extension to further increase velocity and direct the path of the arc closer to the body.

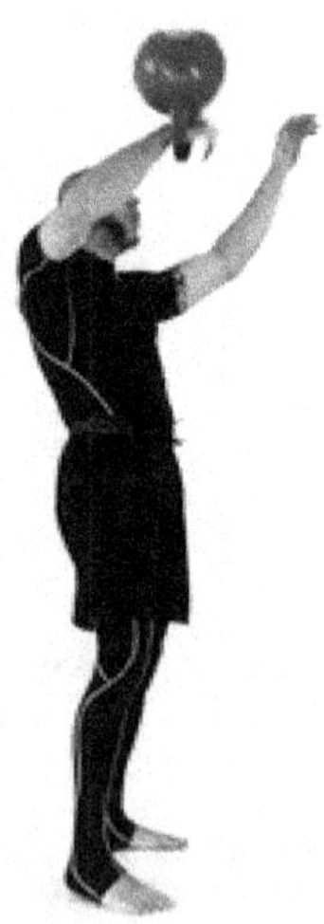

This is what I also call the float. The float is the point where the deceleration jerk takes place, it's the highest point you were able to power the swing and pull. It's not really a float but it sometimes helps the athlete with the understanding that this is the point to let go and insert. If at this stage no hand insertion would happen, then the bell would flop over. Flopping the bell over the fist is something we don't want happening. Flopping of the bell also happens when there is hesitation, the full movement needs to be smooth without any hesitation, the hesitation usually happens at this stage where the insert needs to happen and the bell needs to be guided around the fist.

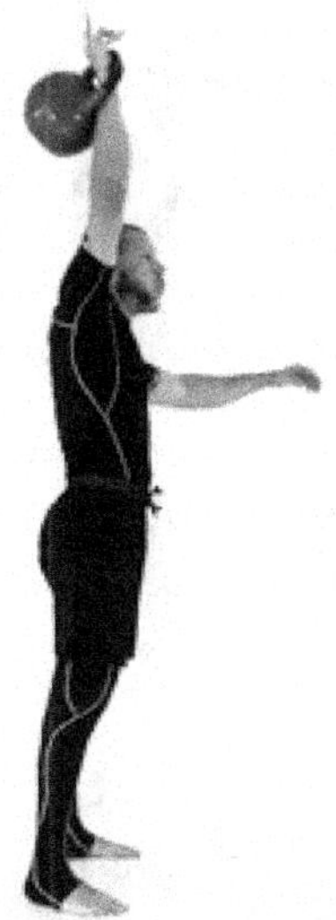

Scoop up the kettlebell and extend the arm overhead.

A good overhead position is where the triceps are active to lock out the elbows, you keep pressing up, not literally, but that's how it should feel. Your shoulder blades are pulled down and slightly together, your chest is semi-firm, and your lats are pulling down to keep the shoulders safe. Side-on all your joints are aligned, wrist, shoulder, hips, knees, and ankles. Your head should be neutral, it will most likely feel like you need to push it forward to keep it neutral, this will depend on your flexibility.

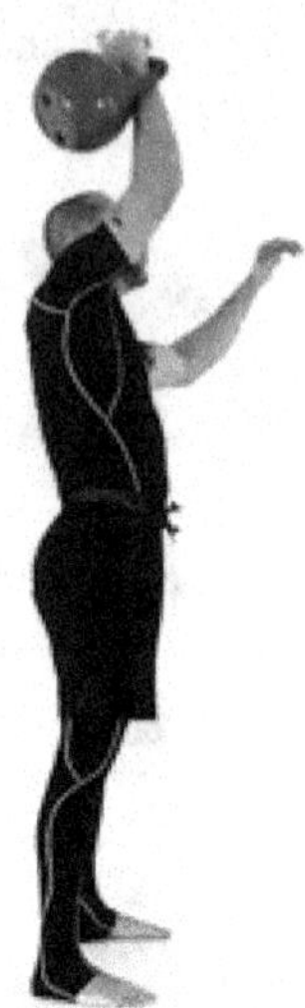

The head is moved back so that the kettlebell can drop straight down and no further movement is required. We want to avoid unnecessary movement. The weight drop in a straight path down, if you were using two kettlebells then the grip changed to a racking safety grip to avoid the fingers getting caught between the handles.

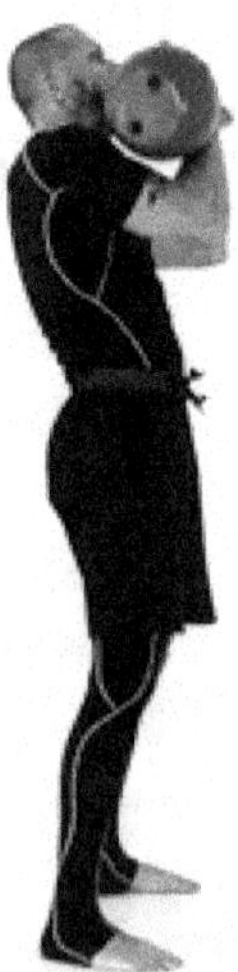

During the drop, the elbows are kept under the weight. With a heavyweight, you can reduce impact through lifting the heels, with an extremely heavyweight you can also use the knees to reduce impact.

A good rack is achieved with the elbows tucked and bells resting in the cradle of the forearm and upper arm.

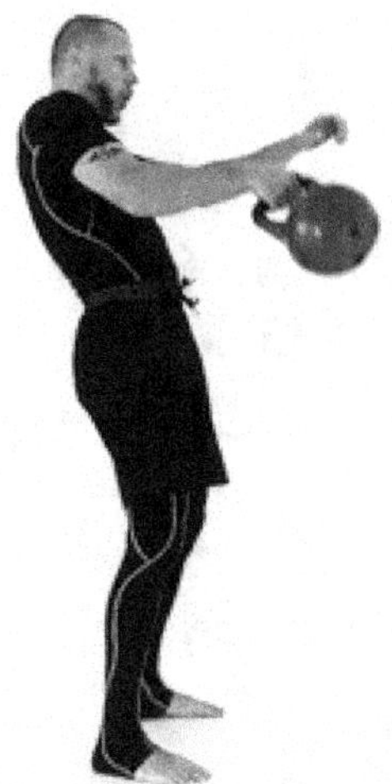

Let the kettlebell drop naturally. Do not cast the bell away from you and follow-through, do the opposite, drop and move away from it. With your upper body moving back you pull out and at the same time are in a better position to control the weight and guide it to the back.

Create hip hyperextension and pull out to catch the kettlebell. Change from loose to hook grip. Come into elbow extension as fast as possible at this stage. Extended elbows will prevent any sudden jerks on the shoulders at a later stage on the drop.

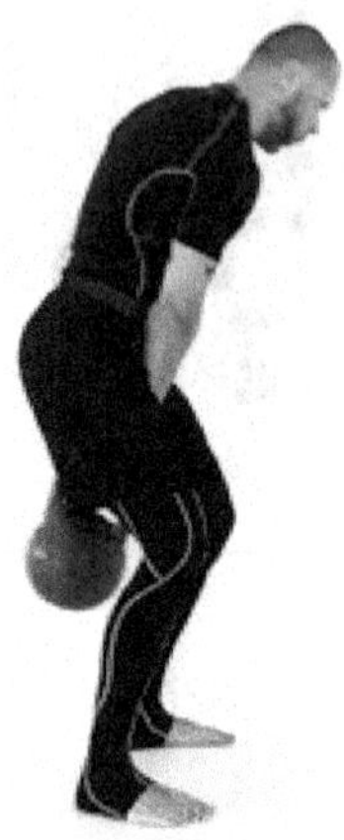

Time to create hip flexion (hip hinge). The kettlebell come through around knee height, the shoulders are still close to being above the ankles at this stage, this is to prevent pressure on the lower back.

At this stage you can perform an insert to assist in reversing the trajectory of the kettlebell smoothly, i.e. you're pushing the kettlebell back and at the same time reduce velocity. The arm can only go so far, so make sure you get the deceleration right and avoid a sudden jerk on the shoulder. You're ready to pull out again. With the pendulum swing, you would perform knee extension to provide more space and let gravity do the work to reverse the trajectory.

On the upswing, you can go against the force, or you can wait and go with the upswing of the kettlebell to help increase velocity.

Velocity can be increased through a direct pull or with a push. With a pull, the arm will be disconnected early on in the upswing, and with a push, the arm will stay connected as long as possible. The longest connection would end after the extend of hip and thoracic hyperextension.

This is just one way of snatching and there are so many variation and changes one can implement for efficiency or other goals that a whole book is devoted the kettlebell snatch, it can be purchased on Cavemantraining.com or Amazon. go.cavemantraining.com/kbe-snatch-book

Bonus videos:
10 Quick Steps To Kettlebell Snatching go.cavemantraining.com/kbe-vid-120
Online Kettlebell Snatch Certification By Cavemantraining™ go.cavemantraining.com/kbe-snatch-vertification
Kings Combo go.cavemantraining.com/kbe-vid-121

Bonus workouts:

30 Minutes Alternating Half Snatch go.cavemantraining.com/kbe-vid-122
The Deadly SIXFOURFOUR EIGHTY go.cavemantraining.com/kbe-vid-123
Kettlebell Snatch Workout go.cavemantraining.com/kbe-vid-124
Snatchery 2.0 WOD go.cavemantraining.com/kbe-vid-125
Kettlebell Workout RAMPAGE go.cavemantraining.com/kbe-vid-126
Kettlebell Workout Nova go.cavemantraining.com/kbe-vid-127
Kettlebell Interval Workout MORTUUS GEMINUS 50 go.cavemantraining.com/kbe-vid-128

Lawnmower Snatch

This is what I named the lawnmower snatch as it resembles the pull of a lawnmower cord. This version of the snatch is great if you have good flexibility and want to put that to the test. You need a good squat with the weight being slightly positioned behind you. The position requires great tension throughout the body to be performed correctly.

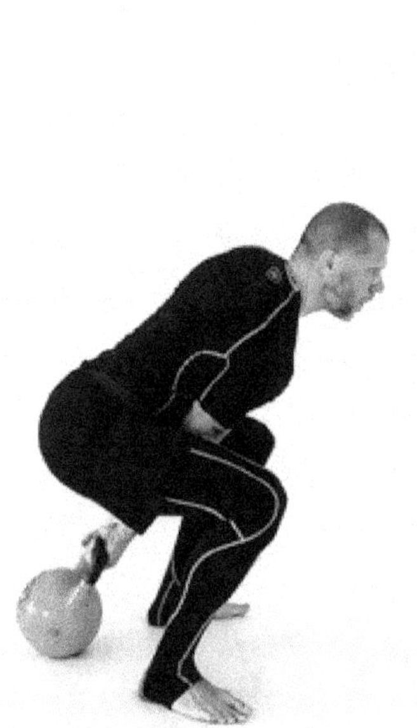
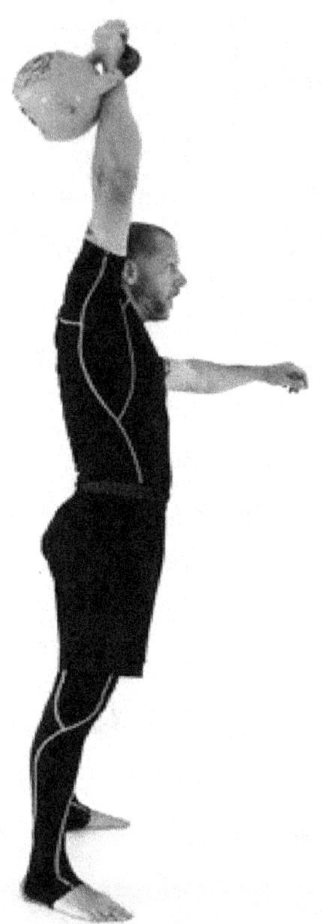

Pendulum Snatch

A pendulum is a weight suspended from a pivot so that it can swing freely.

There are two pendulum concepts in the swing, one relates to your arms, you should never try and shoulder raise the kettlebell during the swing but let them act like a pendulum and move freely. The other is the movement of the swing, it can be a pull or a pendulum, with the first going against resistance, and the second acting upon gravitation and as much as possible like a true pendulum.

It's not a pendulum if your hips are stopping the kettlebell and you're pulling the weight back out, but that doesn't mean it's incorrect, you just need to know when to use one over the other. Do you want to do high or heavy reps or do you want to work your cardiovascular system? Do you want to tax your gluteus maximus as much as possible or do you want to balance it out?

With the pendulum swing, you want to avoid abruptly stopping the kettlebell with your body at the end of the backswing (also cause for bobbing), you can achieve this as best as possible through knee flexion and getting your groin/hips as high as possible. At the endpoint of the backswing you want to let gravity take control and follow along with the hips to accelerate the weight.

The key is to keep your arms connected to the body as long as possible and push forward while the shoulders are coming up, followed by hip and thoracic hyperextension. When working unilaterally you can also pair this with thoracic rotation.

Your thoracic consists of 12 vertebrae, see Th1 to Th12 below. Together with your cervical this is the area that has the most movement in the spine.

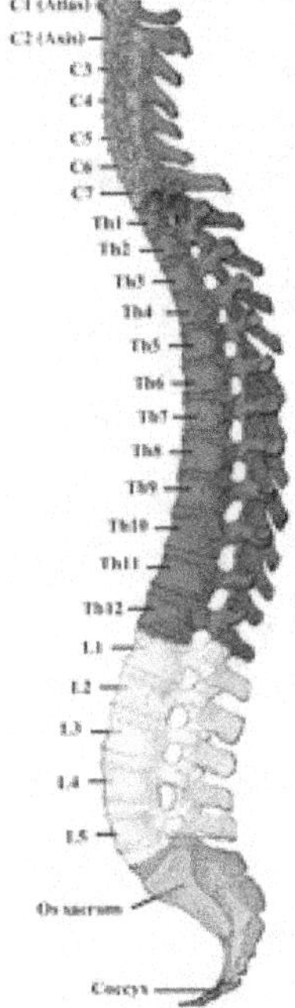

The following sequence of photos is that of the half pendulum snatch. Half because it goes from overhead into racking.

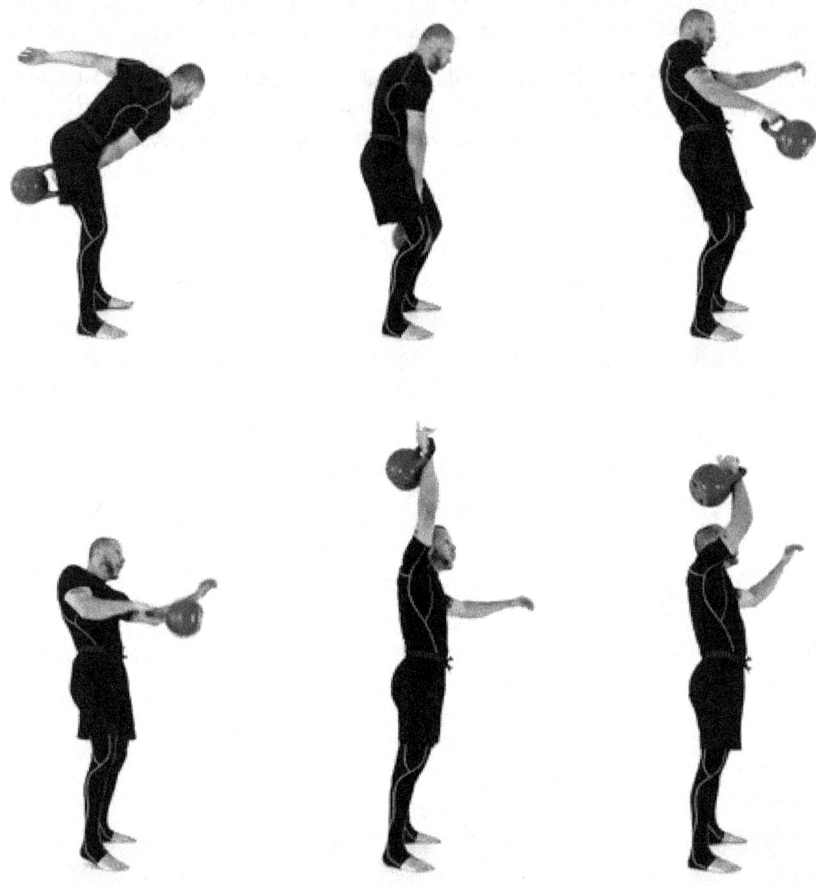

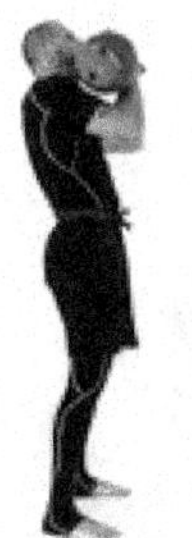 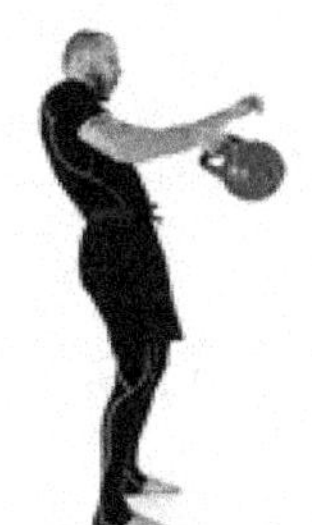 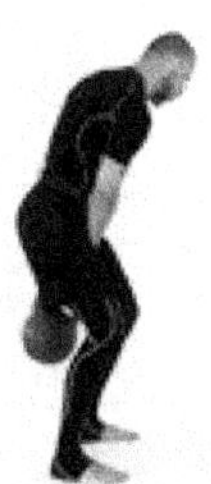 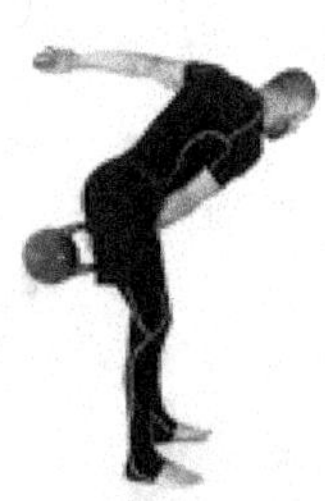

To perform:

1. Ankles, knees, and hips are extended
2. Kettlebell is at the top of the swing
3. Kettlebell is dropping down into the backswing
4. Depending on how high the swing was, the elbow might be flexed or extended
5. The knees flex paired with ankle dorsiflexion as the weight drops past the hips
6. If the elbow was flexed, it should now be extended
7. The bell is guided on the path of the backswing
8. The hips move back to not stop the weight
9. The knees move into extension paired with ankle plantarflexion
10. The shoulders come toward the ground through hip flexion
11. The weight hits the endpoint of the backswing
12. Gravity takes control and the weight starts falling back
13. The hips follow through with knee flexion paired with ankle dorsiflexion
14. The hips are coming into extension
15. All three leg joints move to full extension
16. The torso is upright
17. The movement should be followed by hip and thoracic hyperextension to create a pull for the snatch
18. The kettlebell moves closer to the body
19. As the bell is closer to the body the elbow needs to bend
20. The weight reaches the point where the magnitude of the velocity is 0
21. The motion of the weight changes ass gravity takes control
22. The weight accelerates downwards and is guided into the backswing for another rep

The following sequence of photos is that of the full pendulum snatch AKA pendulum snatch. Full because it drops from overhead straight into the backswing.

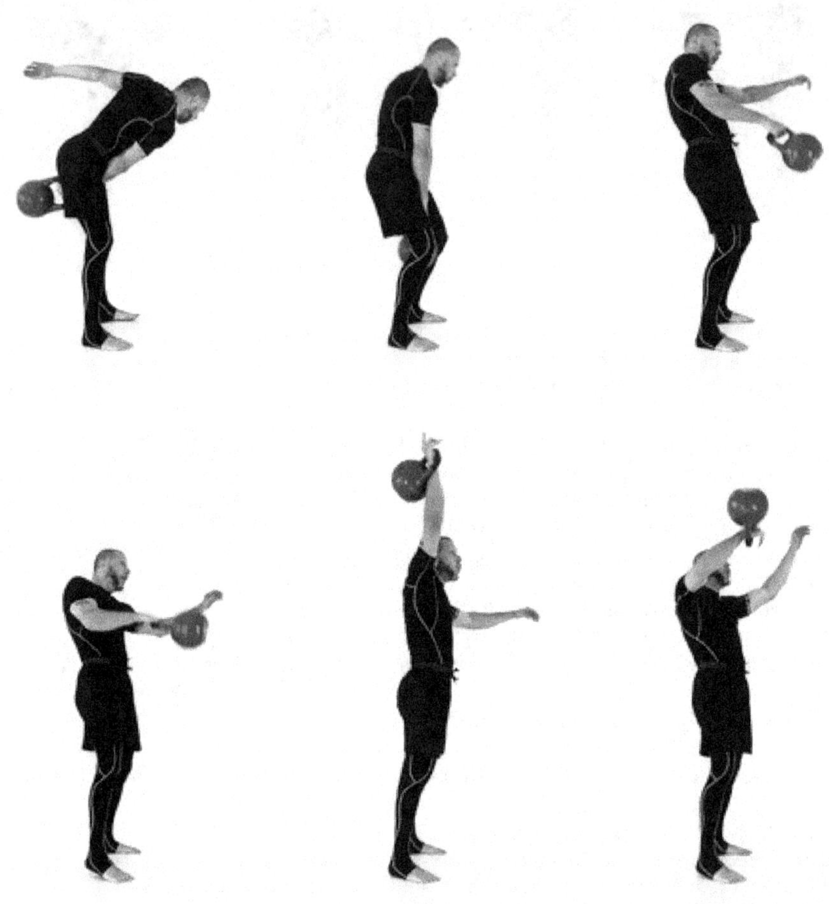

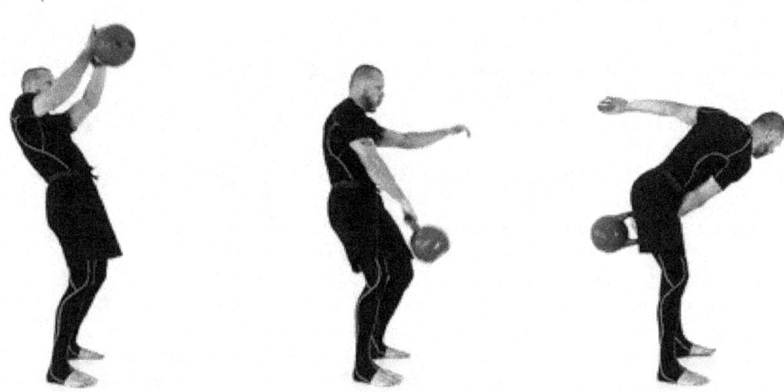

Additional Information

The following sections are additional supporting information for kettlebell training.

Mind-muscle Connection

Movement just happens, you will it and it's done. This is true in a way, some are lucky to have correctly performed a movement so many times it just comes naturally. But throw in a new movement or change an existing movement up and it's a different story.

Mind muscle connection is extremely important, it allows you to recruit more muscles for a movement, the right muscles, and it allows you to isolate muscles for a movement, i.e. purposely not recruit those muscles that <u>can</u> power the movement. It allows you to focus on the muscles you want to work harder and isolate. A great example I'll always go back to is the overhand wide grip pull-up. This exercise can be executed through contraction of many muscles with the main ones being the latissimus dorsi and elbow flexors. Creating elbow flexion when hanging from a bar would bring the shoulders to the bar as the angle in the elbow joints decrease and the hands are not moving away from the bar. Contraction of the lats pulls the elbows toward the hips, i.e. shoulder adduction which in turn will also pull the shoulders to the bar. I repeat again, there are many more muscles involved, like pectoralis major, teres major/minor, infraspinatus, even the triceps brachii long head, etc. but for this example, let's focus on the elbow flexors and lats. Here's where the magic of MMC helps, connect with your elbow flexors and relax them, connect with your lats and contract them, perform the movement with an isolation of the lats and you're truly working on strengthening the lats.

Another example, also with the pull-up. I see many of my athletes start out with not being able to connect with the lats to do a pull-up, they're mainly using the elbow flexors for the pull-up and if not fixed they can quickly develop tendinitis in the elbow flexors. To get them to connect with their lats I will tap the areas which they need to activate and I'll also perform a drill in which the visuals clearly demonstrate whether they're using the lats or elbow flexors.

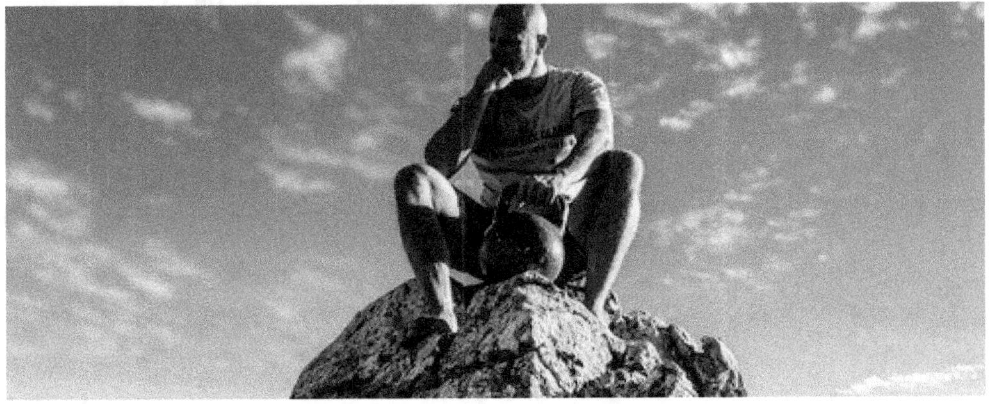

"If an exercise is done with good form, the right muscles do their job automatically." Incorrect. Are the right muscles really doing their work? Are we perhaps talking about an exercise which was progressed to properly with MMC involving all the muscles required, and was that exercise then repeated for high reps over a long period of time? Was that movement and contraction then stored only to be easily recalled and actioned without much thought? I've also been told "but if I squat right now I just do it without much thought", ok, you might be flopping into what you believe is a good squat, or you've done it so many times that yes, you're working with something that has become second nature to do, but… Let's connect with your toes, the balls of your feet, external hip rotation, each of the three gluteals, hip flexors and extensors for pure alignment throughout, let's connect with the muscles around the scapulae for good spinal alignment, and so on. In fact, you do it right now, perform a fast squat as you're used to doing, then **slow down** and pick one of those areas I mentioned and include them through connection. At first you'll need to focus and connect, over time and when performed in high reps the body will get accustomed to it. Progression is again the key here. Slow and with thought. Practice, drill, and repeat, which over time will stick and allow you to go faster with more load.

A great example of connection loss is the toes, with a lot of people it's impossible for them to move their toes separately or at all. This is because the majority of shoes take away the ability to use them through soles that don't easily bend or shoe widths that cramp the toes together which take away the ability to use them for support or balance. Over many years the mind simply does not think about them anymore other than them being ten pieces of flesh hanging from our feet that are nice to decorate with colors. Free them, connect with them, train them, progress them, and over time it becomes natural.

Kettlebell Anatomy

1. Handle
2. Corner(s)
3. Horn(s)
4. Window
5. Bell AKA body
6. Base

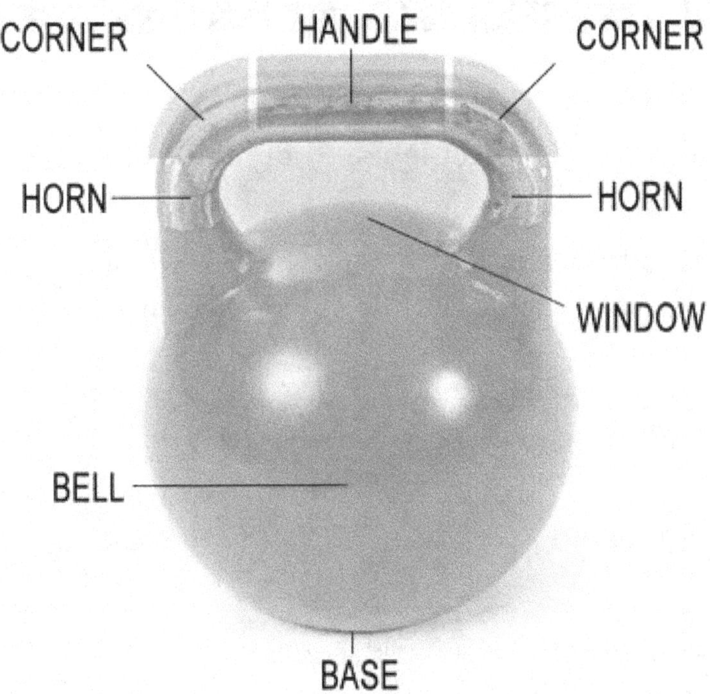

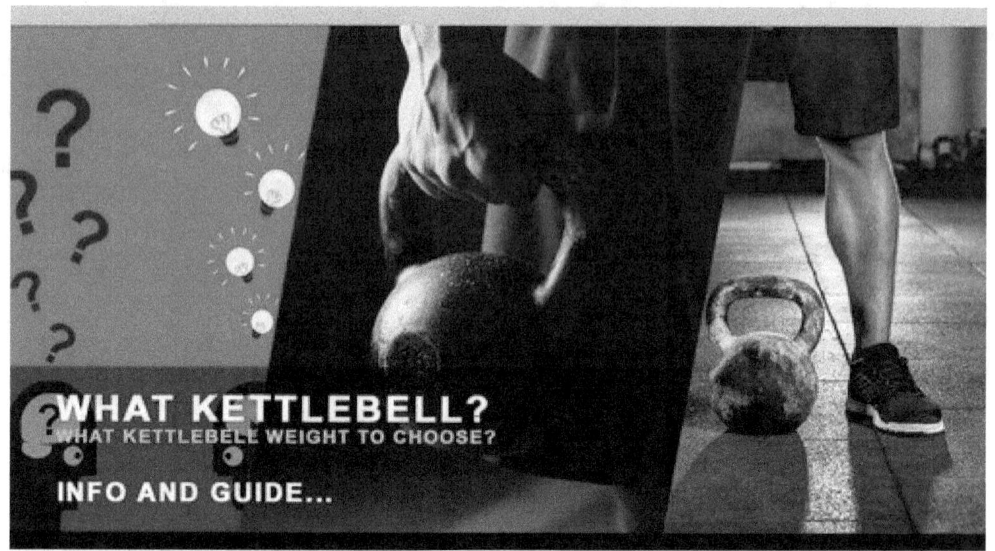

What Weight Kettlebell Should I Start With?

Let's say you're limited to buying one kettlebell, you want to make sure you buy the right kettlebell. **How do you decide what kettlebell weight to choose?**

Kettlebells are not cheap, so you want to make sure you buy the right weight, which will allow you to get the most out of your one kettlebell. Here are some tips to start thinking about what kettlebell weight to choose.

Goals?

What are your goals, why are you buying a kettlebell?

- Lose weight/fat loss
- Gain overall strength
- Become flexible
- Increase cardiovascular endurance
- Etc.

Based on those answers you can compile the exercises you'll mainly want to be doing. Performing a racked squat with a kettlebell is completely different from a ballistic swing, or overhead reverse lunge.

Are you going to be performing high reps, or low reps, swinging 20, 50, 100 or more, or in sets of 6 to 12? If you can handle a 24kg swing, that doesn't mean it's the right weight to use for high volume or endurance. You'll want to go at least 1/3 lower to what your submax is.

If you're mainly going to be doing slow lifts and carries like, deadlifts, farmer walks, racked walks, goblet squats, racked squats, and even some double-arm chest presses etc. you can go considerably higher with the weight. Let's say you would get a 16kg if you were going to swing a lot, then you could easily get a 24 to 28kg for these types of exercises.

If you want to work on endurance or cardio, you'll be doing a higher volume, if you want to work on strength, hypertrophy, then you'll be doing lower volume.

Current State?

What is your current state, how strong, flexible, fit are you? If you've never touched a weight in your life before, then you'll need a different weight than someone who has been going to the gym for years.

Are you very inflexible? If so, this will also affect the weight you choose. You'll run more risk of injury if you're inflexible, hence you'll need to reduce the weight and focus on flexibility more.

Experience?

Have you already got some experience with lifting barbells, dumbbells, etc.? If so, it will be easier to understand some of the concepts in kettlebell training, hence, you'll be safer, so you can increase the weight you choose. But, you should still take into consideration that the kettlebell has a different weight distribution than the barbell or dumbbell, this will make the kettlebell feel much heavier, i.e. if you're pressing a 30kg dumbbell 1RM, you'll need to subtract 4kg or more for a kettlebell, as you won't be able to transfer the exact amount to a kettlebell.

Have you got no experience what so ever with a kettlebell or any other weight? You should seriously consideration this, and start at the low end. Safety first.

Guide

Following is a guide on what kettlebell weight to choose, however, you should consider all the points above first and make your own informed decision.

Lots of overhead work	Male		Female	
	Low Volume	High Volume	Low Volume	High Volume
Never done anything overhead	8 to 12kg	8 to 10kg	8kg	8kg
Mediocre with overhead work	12 to 16kg	12kg	12kg	10kg
Do overhead work in the gym regularly	16 to 20kg	16kg	16kg	12kg
Lots of slow lifts	**Male**		**Female**	
	Low Volume	High Volume	Low Volume	High Volume
Never done any slow lifts	16kg	12kg	12kg	10kg
Mediocre with slow lifts	20 to 24kg	16kg	18kg	16kg
Do slow lifts in the gym regularly	24 to 32kg	20kg	24kg	20kg
Lots of ballistic work	**Male**		**Female**	
	Low Volume	High Volume	Low Volume	High Volume
Never done anything ballistic	12 to 16kg	12kg	12kg	10kg
Mediocre with ballistic work	16 to 20kg	16kg	16kg	14kg
Do ballistic work in the gym regularly	20 to 24kg	20kg	20kg	16kg

Still not sure? Buy an online assessment, discuss your goals, submit your video, get feedback, and a recommendation.

Which Kettlebell to Choose and Why?

I'm a great advocate for competition kettlebells, even when not used for Kettlebell Sport. That said, I'll provide as much information about the different kettlebells available, so you can make your own decision.

If you're just starting with kettlebell training, you'll want to start with something light, so that you can focus on form and technique. Starting with a weight that is too heavy will compromise your form and technique, and potentially cause injury.

Differences:

- Handle diameter
- Handle shape
- Window diameter
- Base diameter
- Bell dimension
- Weight
- Colour
- Coat
  - Neoprene
  - Rubber
  - Vinyl
  - Powder
- Material
  - Steel
  - Iron
- Filling
  - Sand
  - Water
  - Hollow

Competition Kettlebells AKA Pro Grade Kettlebells, Sport Kettlebells, Girya Sport Kettlebell

Classic Kettlebells AKA Iron-cast Kettlebells

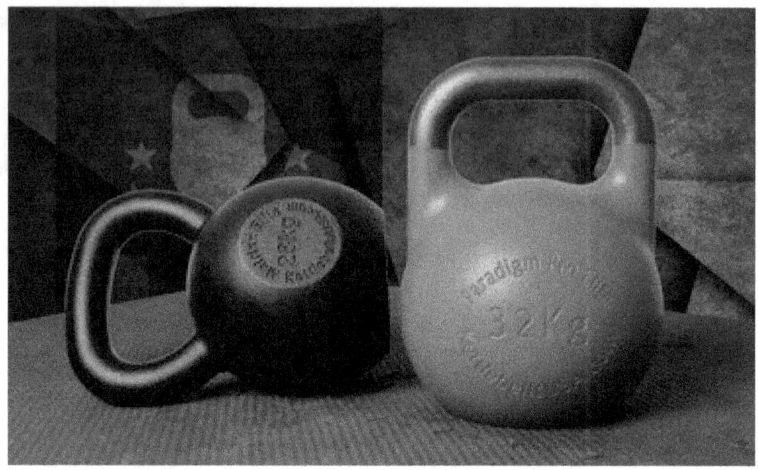

Cast-iron versus Steel Competition Kettlebell

Classic Kettlebells are less expensive than the Competition Kettlebells.

As mentioned earlier, my preference is the Competition Kettlebell and the reason for that is the competition kettlebell remains the same size, no matter what weight you work with; whether it's an 8kg or 24kg, the size of the kettlebell remains the same. This is a great feature because there is no need to get used to different shapes and sizes when you go up in weight. Furthermore, the base of the comp kettlebell is a lot wider, allowing you to do things like burpee deadlifts, renegade rows, and other exercises where you need to place your weight on the kettlebell - a narrow base has the potential for the bell to topple over and cause wrist injury. I find it difficult to find comfortable positions with the classic kettlebells, especially the lighter weight.

Rubber, neoprene, and vinyl-coated kettlebells are more suitable for surfaces that scratch or chip easily. Vinyl is harder and more resistant to damage than rubber. Neoprene is softer than both rubber and vinyl, which increases comfort. All that said, I've not had good experience with these type of coated kettlebells myself.

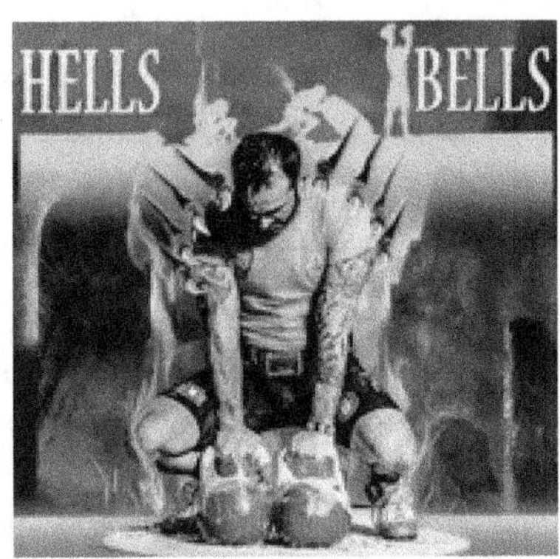

David Keohan

International Kettlebell Colour Standard for Competition Kettlebells:

Weight in Kilos	Weight in Pounds	Colour
8	17.6 (order)	Pink
12	26.4 (order)	Blue
16	35.2 (order)	Yellow
20	44.0 (order)	Purple
24	52.8 (order)	Green
28	61.6 (order)	Orange
32	70.4 (order)	Red
36	79.2 (order)	Grey
40	88.0 (order)	White
44	96.8 (order)	Silver
48	105.6	Gold

There are also weights in between (for example, 10 kg, 14 kg, and so on), and these are usually colored with a different shade of the neighboring weight, or defined by a black band on the handle.

What Weight to Choose?

The weight you choose for training depends on your goals and what exercises you will primarily be doing with it, in addition to your current strength. If we're talking primarily about double-arm swings done by absolute beginners, I'd suggest 8kg or less for children, 10kg to 12kg for adolescents, 12kg for women, and 14 to 16kg for men.

For overhead pressing, I suggest at least 4 to 6kg less than mentioned for the swings above. For chest pressing, 2 to 4kg less, as most people are stronger with chest presses compared to overhead presses.

For rowing with the focus being on the rear deltoids, I suggest the same weight as for swings or even slightly more weight. For rows that focus more on the middle of the back, I suggest the same weight as for overhead presses.

For deadlifts, squat style, I suggest the same as swings or more, and possibly even double kettlebells. For deadlifts hip hinge, I recommend the same as swings or slightly less.

That covers the basic exercises. If you're talking about any other exercise, you've already progressed and are more than likely able to make an informed decision on what weight to use.

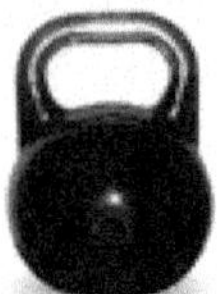 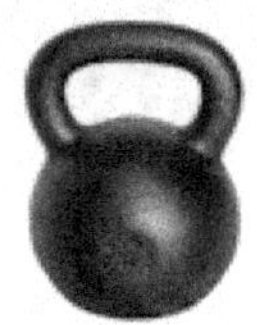 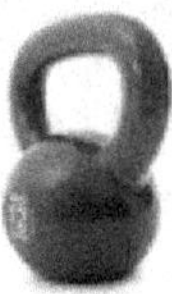 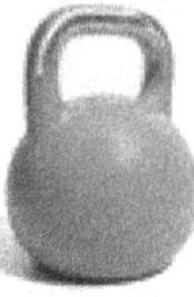

Where to Buy Kettlebells Online

Out of the many places to buy kettlebells online, you'll see the following names and brands pop up the most: Amazon, Kettlebell Kings, DragonDoor/RKC, Onnit, Agatsu, Ader, Kettlebells USA.

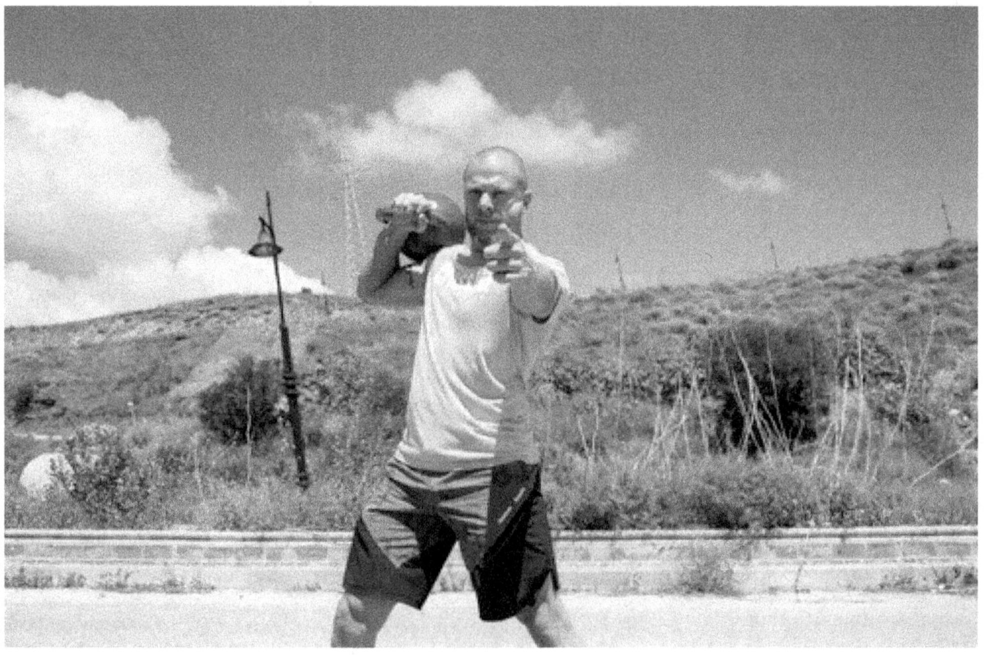

Kettlebell Grips

There are many different types of kettlebell grips you will need to employ during kettlebell training, the following are photos and basic explanations of what each different grip is used for. If you enrolled in one of our free or paid online kettlebell courses you will see these different grips referred to.

Important: with each grip, there are only one or two exercises listed to get a general idea across, but in most cases, there are many more than those listed. Grips might differ slightly across kettlebells, as the width of the handle increases with some of the classic kettlebells when the weight goes up.

Along your kettlebell journey, you will find that different associations or organizations will use different grips for different exercises, and as long as it works and is safe, there is nothing wrong with it.

For illustration purposes, a competition kettlebell is used, which changes in weight but not in size.

Note that these are **not** barbell grips, as the names might be the same, the technique is not.

"excellent document and the content is highly accurate"
~ Valerie Pawlowski World Champion Kettlebell Lifting

General Information

The following rules and tips apply in general to most kettlebell grips. A grip on the kettlebell handle or horns should almost never be tight, it should be as loose as possible without losing grip of the kettlebell and conserving as much grip strength without burning out the muscles.

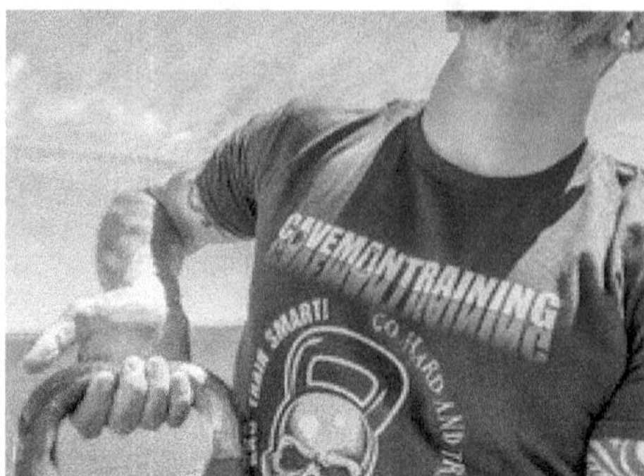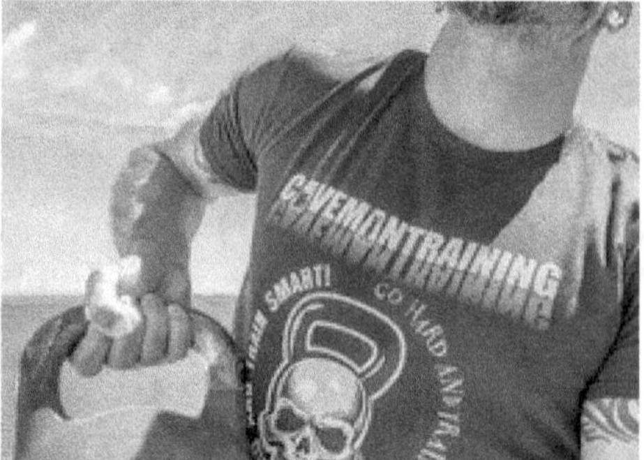

Loose versus tight grip

Blisters usually occur when the skin is folded within the grip, especially when using heavy weights or doing high volume reps. Try and slide your fingers around the handle or horns while keeping skin folds from occurring and then close the grip. Another cause for blisters is friction, avoid friction by proper kettlebell guidance (which you'll learn in our courses).

Ripped calluses usually occur when there is friction within the palms, biggest culprit is kettlebell bobbing, to prevent the kettlebell from bobbing search for my article online 'kettlebell swing insert', the insert prevents the kettlebell from doing a full pendulum which is usually causing abrupt stopping of the kettlebell.

"You should look at it like this. If you're making the pendulum movement and let the bell go where it wants to go, it abruptly gets stopped by your body, i.e. your arms hit your thighs or whatever part of the body, the bell will want to keep going, this is creating the friction in your hands, on high reps or heavyweight this will cause blisters.

To fix, think about directing the weight to the back, create a deep insert, think first part of the swing PENDULUM and then bang, INSERT. Direct the weight to the back. Hope that helps."

The most **common grip** and **transition** are that from hook grip to loose grip which occurs during the clean and rack, the hook grip is also used for single-arm swings and snatches, the second most common grip is the double hand grip which is used for double arm swings.

This transition is one that beginners should focus on, the need to want to hold the kettlebell handle tight, and perform no transition is high with beginners. This is such an important concept that everyone should spend a lot of time on until they get it right. I can highly recommend performing assisted cleans to work on this.

Why should you learn about grips?

It is important to know and understand kettlebell grips for efficiency and being able to work the muscles intended for the exercise in question. Employing an incorrect grip can mean pain; being uncomfortable; cause for injury; exhausting grip, forearm, biceps or shoulder muscles and losing focus on the muscles targeted with a specific exercise.

Why use different grips?

If you're asking this question, then you're asking the right question because knowing a lot of grips is cool, but knowing why you would change grip or use one over the other is even cooler and the part you should really understand.

During kettlebell training, you employ different grips to make certain exercises more efficient, but you also change grips to increase difficulty and challenge other muscle groups. Sometimes when your training gets stale you might even employ a different grip to please the mind.

While knowing kettlebell grips and when to employ them is important and one of the kettlebell fundamentals, the second most important thing you should start looking into is racking a kettlebell. It might seem insignificant, but a lot hinges on how you rack your kettlebell, in fact, some people give up on kettlebell training because they can't get comfortable in the racking position or can't find the proper position for the bell to rest.

Search Google for 'Cavemantraining Kettlebell Racking' to start learning about this next topic in kettlebell fundamentals.

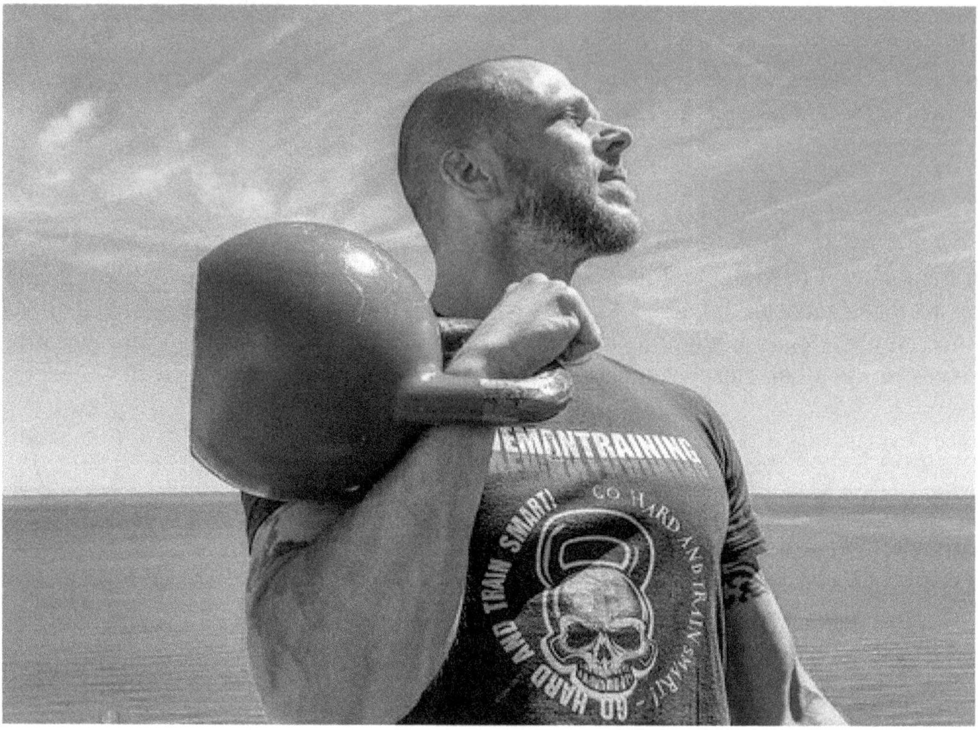

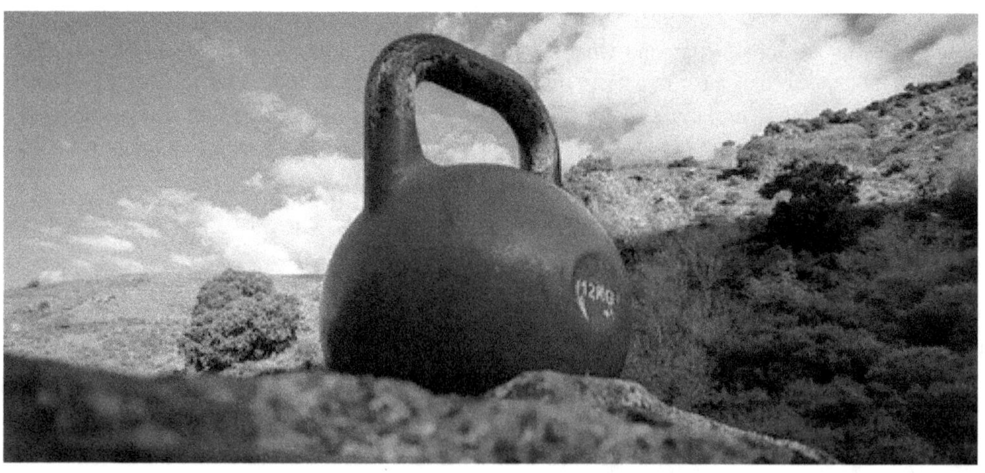

I invite you to watch a video on our YouTube channel which demonstrates several kettlebell clean transitions into different grips go.cavemantraining.com/mkg-vid-1

45-Degree Angle

In grips employed for **racking** or **pressing**, the handle should be positioned at a 45-degree angle within the palm, one corner positioned between the thumb and index finger, and the other corner is past the heel of the palm. The reason for this position is to keep the wrist straight and hand in line with the forearm, this will avoid pressure on the wrist. A bent wrist means there is a kink in the line through which power will be lost during pressing plus the cause for potential injury.

When working with a light kettlebell this might not be so noticeable, but when working with heavier kettlebells the pressure can be enormous, cause damage to the wrist and/or prevent you from being able to press the kettlebell up.

When people first start training with a kettlebell, you'll find that they employ the broken wrist grip to relieve the pressure that the bell provides on the forearm, this is especially so for new people who are not used to this pressure. You should take the person aside and have them play with the grip, handle position and bell positioning until they feel ok with the pressure of the kettlebell being in the correct position. You should also explain that it's quite normal to experience some mild discomfort until the area is more conditioned.

See illustrations below for correct 45-degree handle angle in the palm.

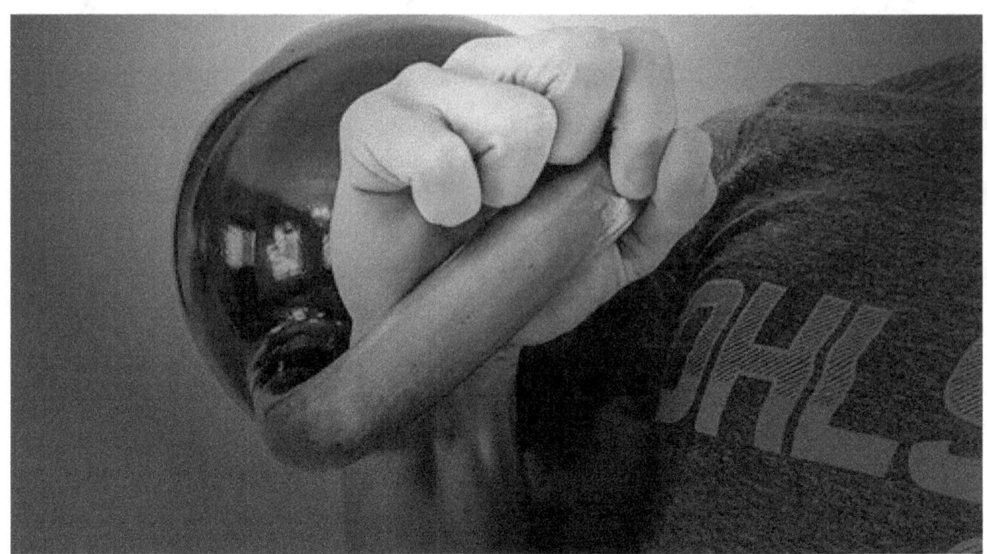

Correct 45° angle of the handle within the palm

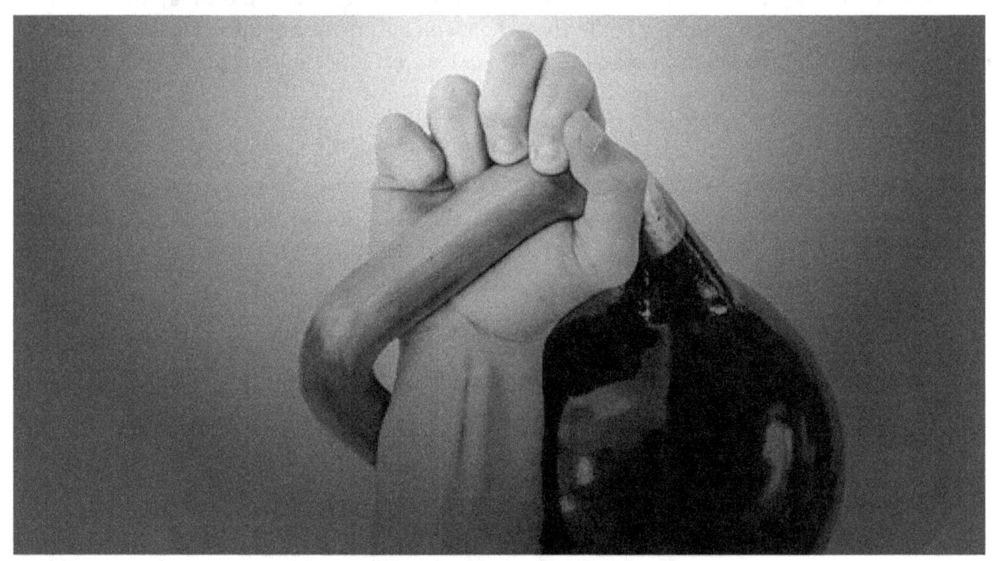

Correct 45° angle of the handle within the palm

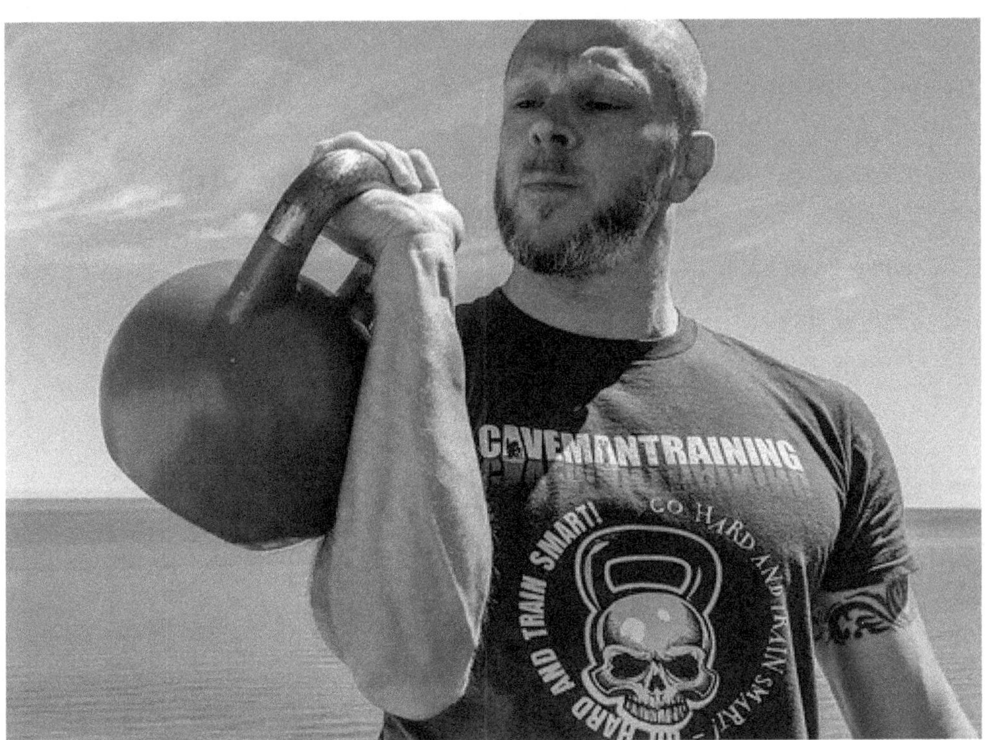

Handle incorrectly positioned within the palm, AKA "broken wrist"
note that the left corner is not over the heel of the palm

Grip Categories

Grips can be categorized in the following categories:

- Pressing grips
- Racking grips
- Lifting grips
- Ballistic grips
- Juggling grips

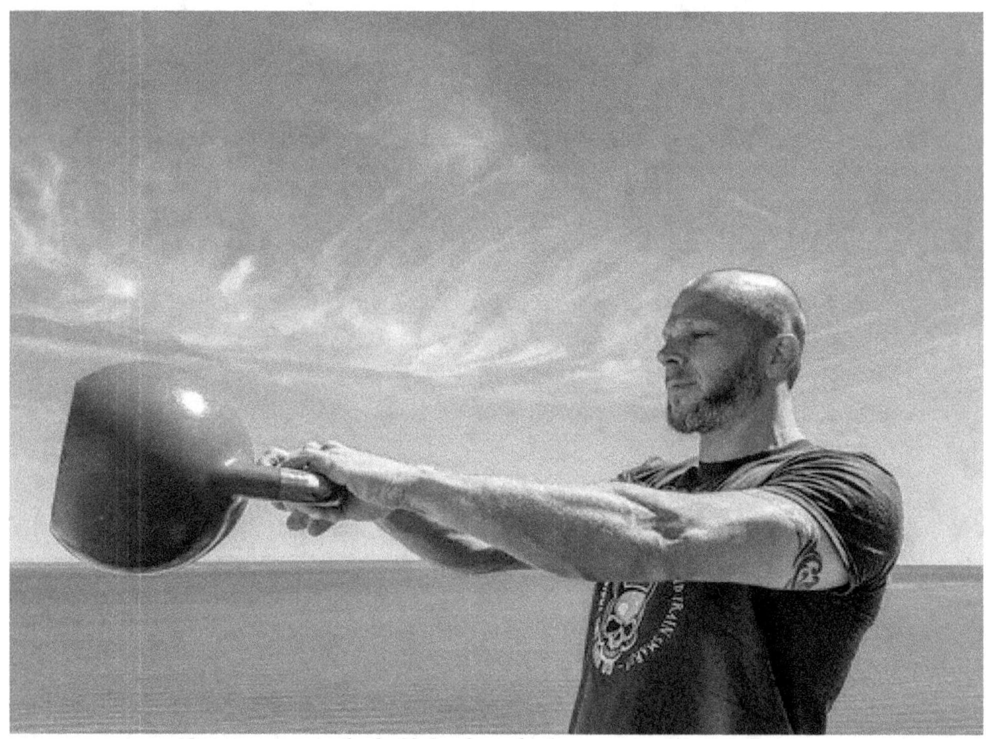

Most common grip, the double hand grip for the conventional kettlebell swing

Broken Wrist Grip—incorrect grip

As the name implies, this is not a grip you'll want to employ. It's named so because the straight-line your arm and palm should be in is broken. A correct kettlebell grip is one of the main things to focus on when you start kettlebell training. You have to get it right, take some time away from everyone and take a light kettlebell, play with it, move it around till you find the two or three points in racking where the weight should rest. The resting points are; around the heel of the palm; on the forearm; and against the biceps when in cradle racking position.

When your wrist is not straight/neutral in racking or overhead position, all the weight is pulling down on your wrist. Most people employ this incorrect grip because they might feel less pressure on the forearm, however, one should take the time to find the right resting points to maintain a neutral wrist. The second cause for an incorrect grip/insert is a tight grip and not opening up during the clean for a proper hand insert.

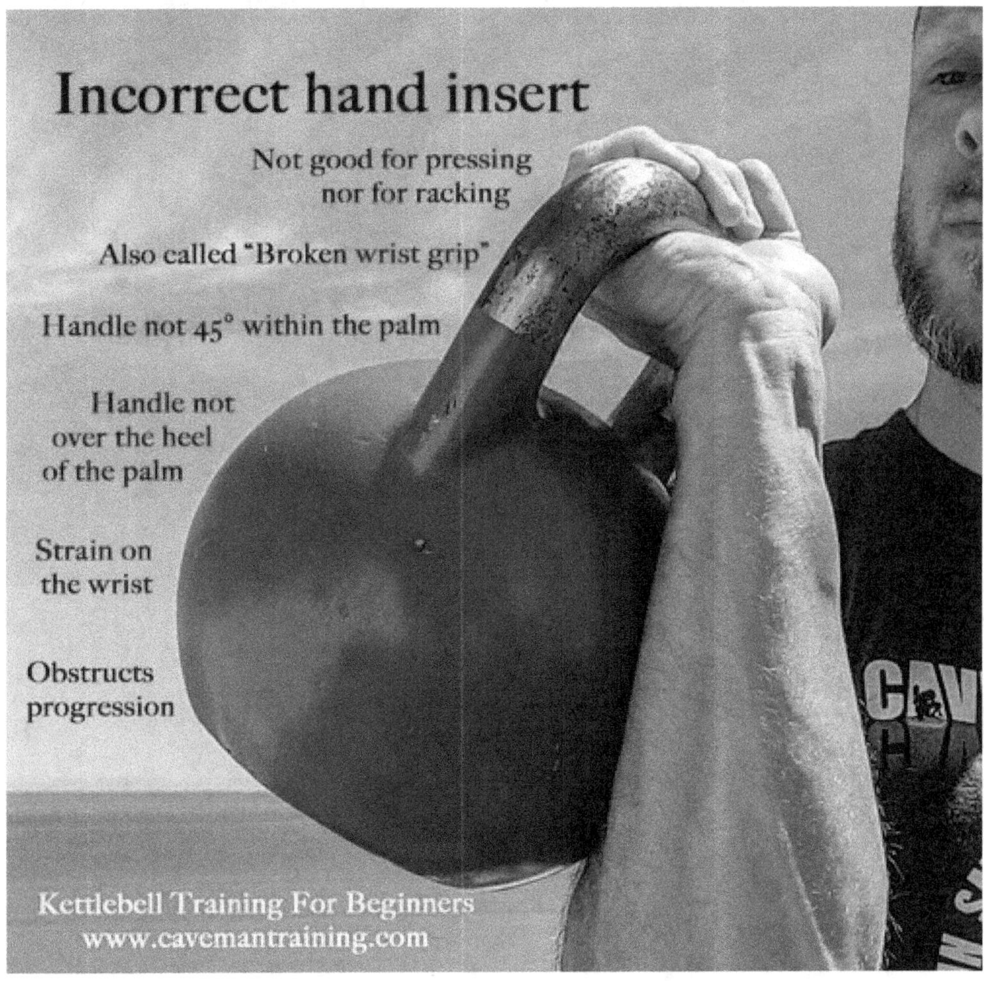

The above photo can be saved/shared on Facebook from the following link:

go.cavemantraining.com/mkg-link-1

The photo below can be saved/shared on Facebook from:

go.cavemantraining.com/mkg-link-2

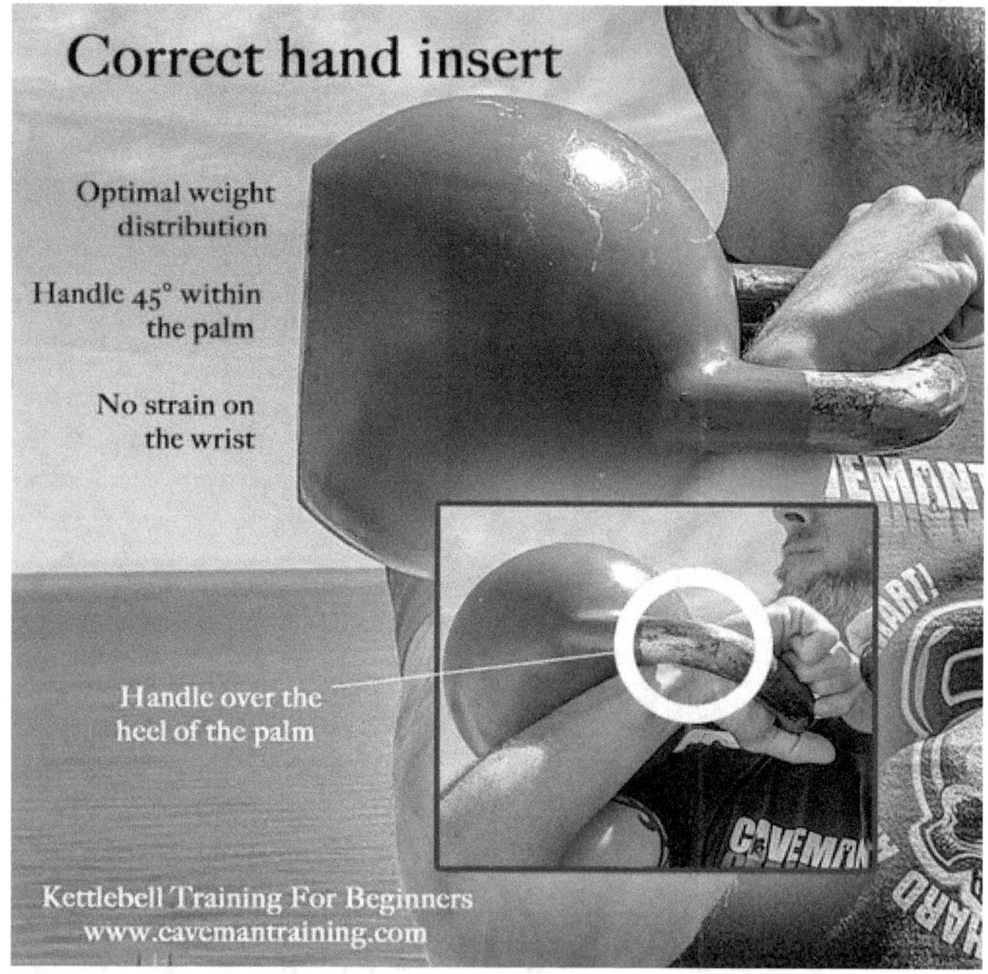

Without further ado, let's dive deep into the kettlebell grips.

Double Hand Grip

Grip: two hands, four fingers closed around the handle placed on the corners or horns depending on hand size and thumbs loose.

Ideal for: double-arm swings and deadlifts

This grip is mostly used for doing double arm swings and deadlifts. Like with most grips, do not turn this into a tight grip, keep some space for the handle to move freely without causing friction. This grip should loosen up at the top part of the swing to stop the grip from burning out. You will have eight fingers around the handle, with big hands your fingers might feel squashed when doing high volume reps, pay particular attention to the ring fingers at high volume reps as they'll be prone to blisters.

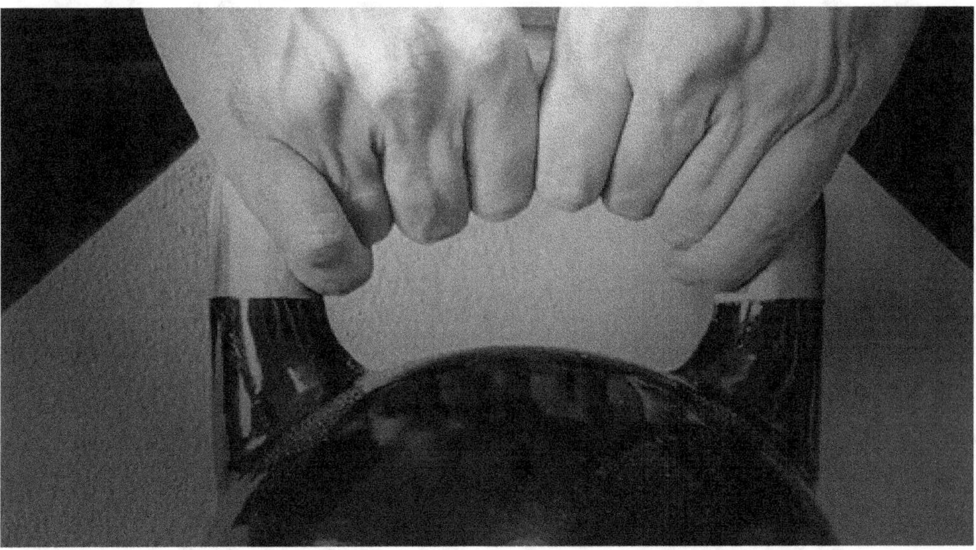

The grip can be employed with both of the pinkies positioned within the horns *(pictured above)* or over the horns *(pictured further below under the Closed Double Hand Grip)*.

Swan Grip

This grip is used primarily in rowing drills and pulling or front holding movements.

Grasping with fingers mostly straight in a beak like hold over top of kettlebell with arm bent at wrist and elbow in "S" like position, as that of swan neck, with emphasis on squeeze of fingers and strong forearm engagement this grip works tremendous grip strength for massive finger and forearm recruitment.

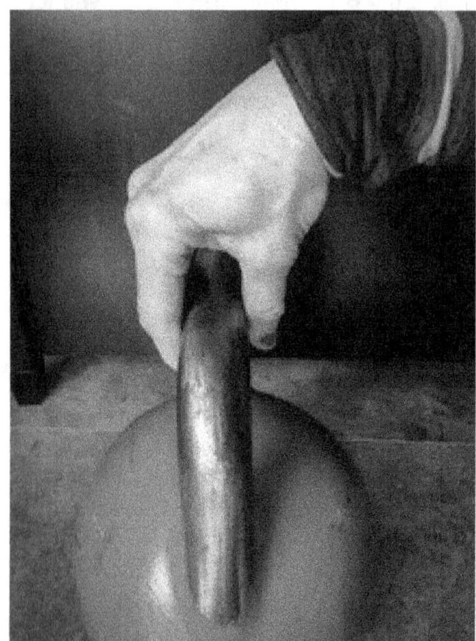
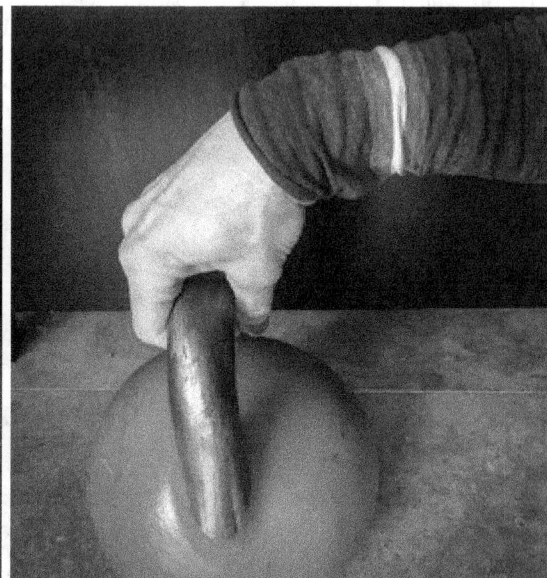

Swan grip

OK Grip (AKA 2 or 3 Finger Grip)

With thumb and first finger (and middle for 3) in an 2 finger lock wrap around handle. Remaining 3 fingers are off or relaxed (2 off on the ok 3 hold) away from handle.

Useful for carries, swings, clean or row. The thumb and first finger are the most important to primary grip strength. Working with these variations puts attention on the longer lasting strength to hang on to the fullest extent especially digging out on final Snatches.

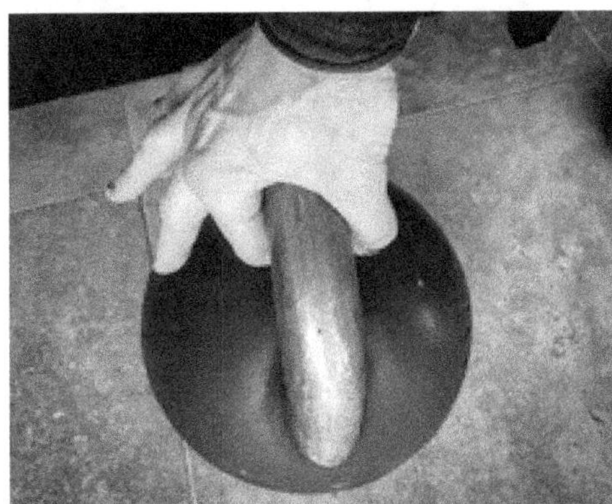 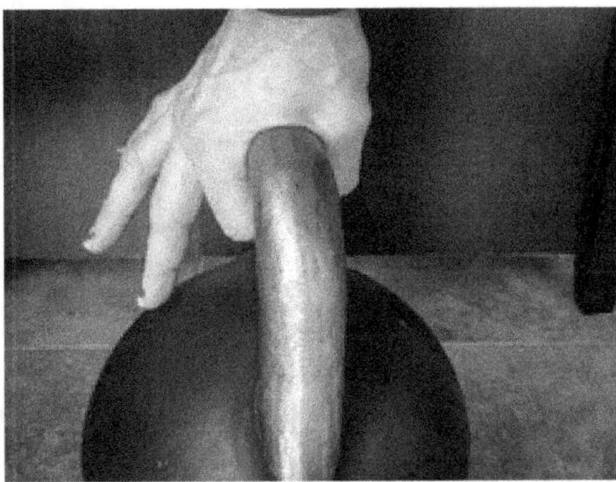

Ok grip
Thanks to Valerie Pawlowski for the photos and information.

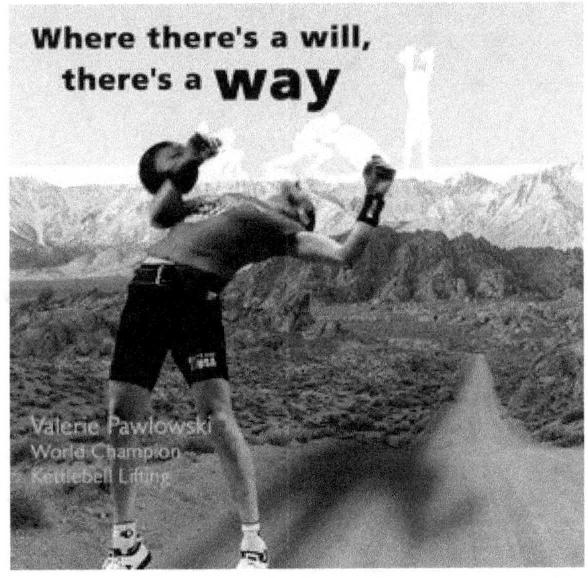

Double Hand Corkscrew Grip

Grip: same as the double hand grip but with the horns between the pinkie and ring fingers.

Ideal for: double-arm swings and American swings

This is a grip I've started using when doing heavy high volume swings during the **Caveman Kettlebells 28 Day Swing Challenge**, which I like to call the Double Hand Corkscrew Grip because it's very similar to a grip on a corkscrew, when holding a corkscrew, the screw itself will be positioned between the middle finger and ring finger, but with the kettlebell the horn will be positioned between the ring finger and pinkie. Everything from the Double Hand Grip transfers to this grip. I like to use this grip to switch it up, but also because I have big hands and usually need to put my pinkies over the handles with the Double Hand Grip, with this grip I feel that my fingers are less squashed. It is very important to wrap your pinkies around the horn to prevent them from getting caught in your clothes during the swing. This grip also provides more stability at the top of the American swing and helps prevent skin tears on the outside of the pinkie.

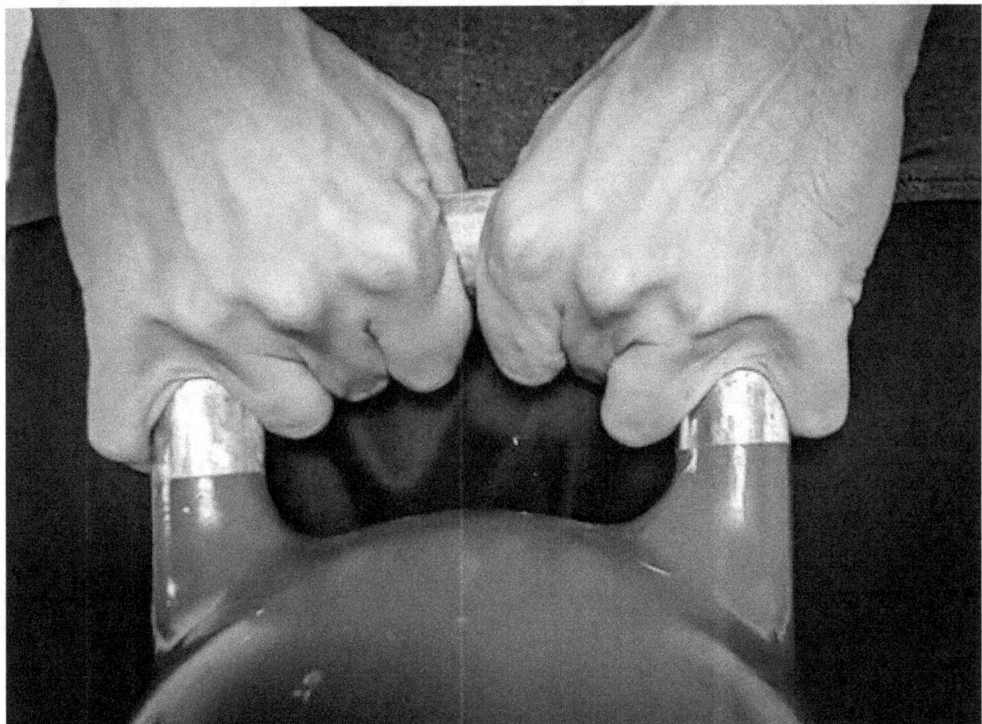

Double hand corkscrew grip

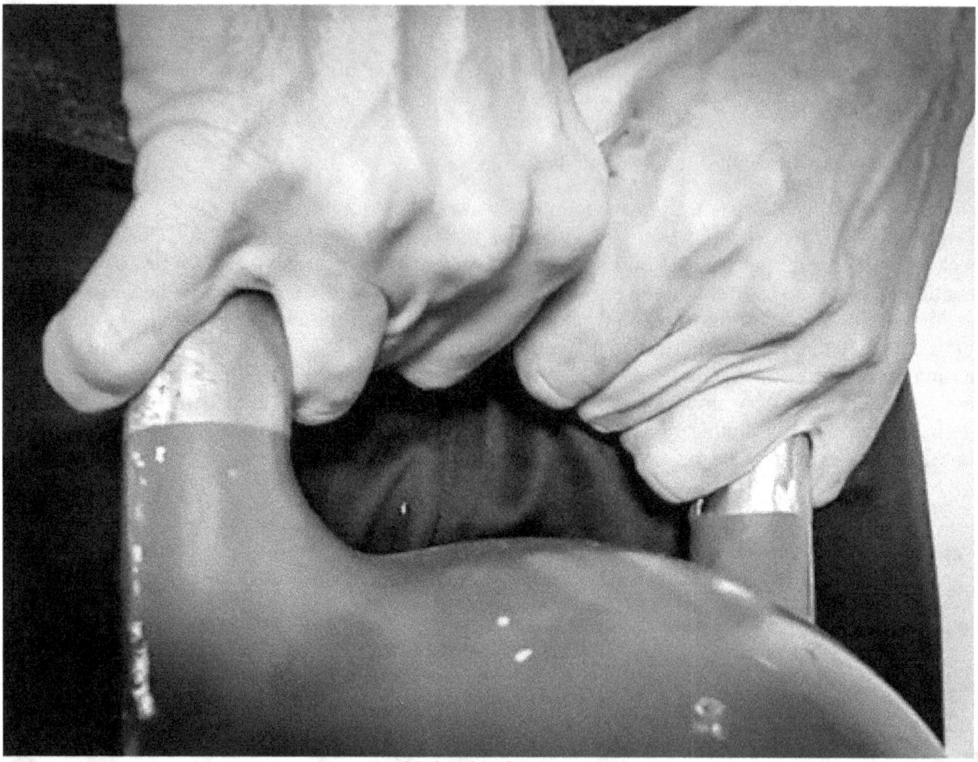

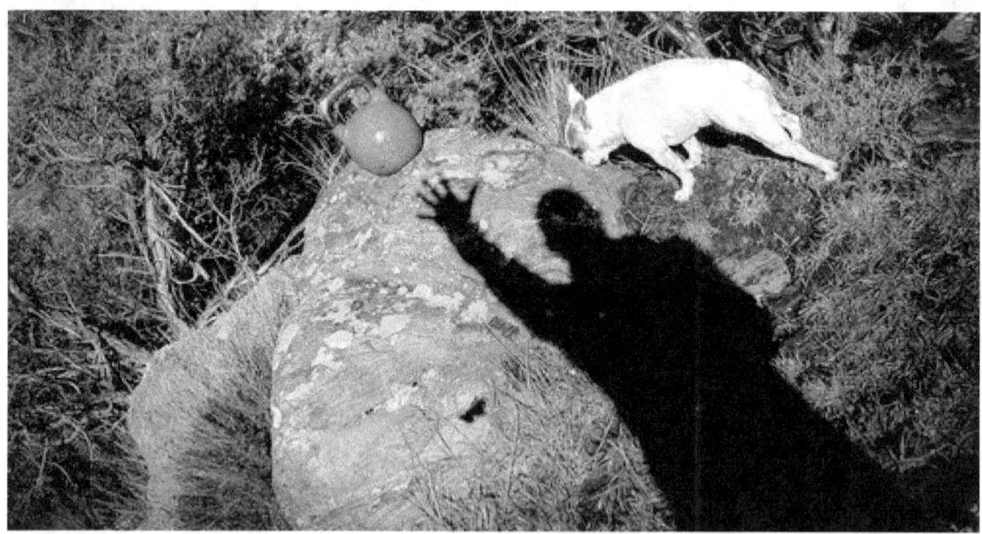

Double hand corkscrew grip

Closed Double Hand Grip

Handle: two hands, four fingers and thumbs locking the index finger down, or locking both the index and middle finger down. Can also be with the pinkies over the horns as illustrated below, in which case it becomes, three fingers plus lock.

Ideal for: double-arm swings, deadlifts

Everything from the Double Hand Grip transfers to this grip, the difference is that the thumbs are locking over the index fingers, this grip is for using extremely heavy weights, or high volume swings and the grip is giving up. The lock is also employed to relieve some tension from the forearms. The lock might also be possible with one thumb two fingers. Note: this grip might not be possible with thicker handles.

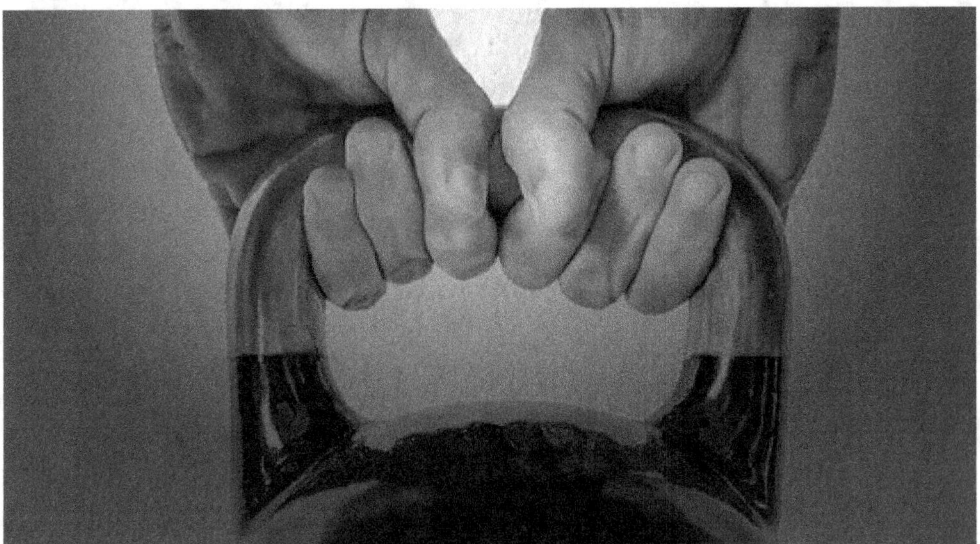

Closed double hand grip

Hook Grip (AKA Overhand Grip)

Handle: one hand, four fingers and thumb loose

Ideal for: down-phase of most ballistic movements, dead clean

With this grip, the handle is positioned within the fingers which are bend, used when the Kettlebell travels downwards for single arm swings and downward phase of snatches. Note that the thumb can move over to the other side of the handle *(but not locking finger)* and the hand is positioned closer to one side of the handle.

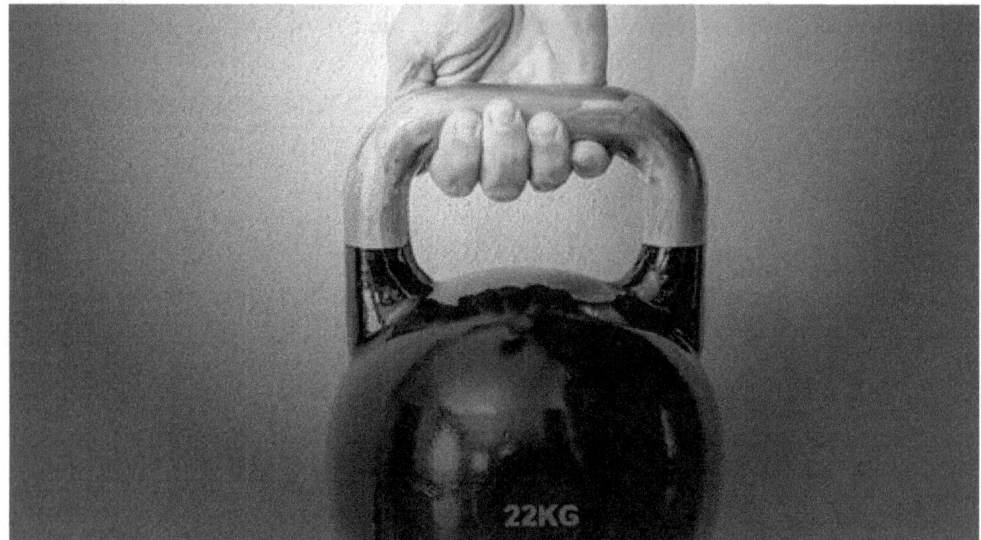

Closed Hook Grip (AKA C grip)

Handle: one hand, four fingers and thumb locking the index finger down, or both the index and middle finger

Ideal for: single-arm swings, snatch, dead clean

This grip is the same as the Hook Grip apart from there being a finger lock with the thumb over forefinger. The lock provides a better grip but also releases tension on the forearms and fingers. If you experience fingers cramps, forearms pains or soreness, try switching to a closed hook grip. Issues arise especially when just starting out with training or when doing high volume reps without implementing a closed grip.

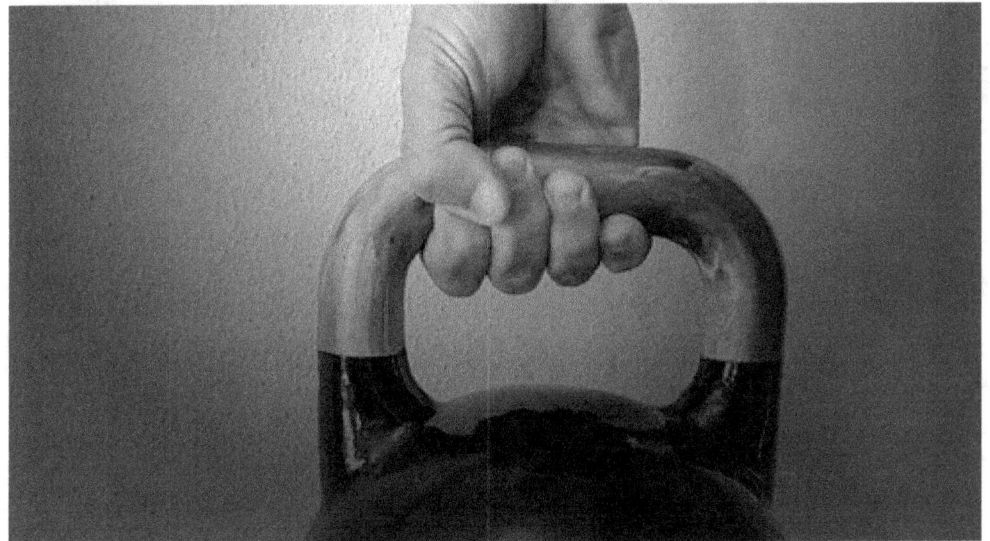

Racking Grip

This is the common grip employed in racking position with a closed but relaxed fist, fingers gently resting on the handle. If you work with two kettlebells you should look at employing the racking safety grip.

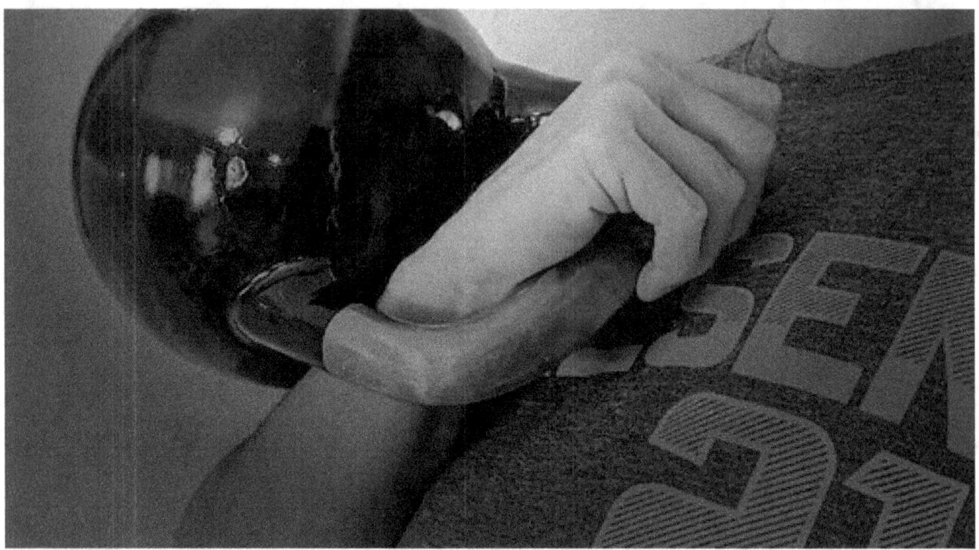

Racking is important for resting, pressing, squatting and all require a different type of rack. Search Google for 'Cavemantraining Kettlebell Racking' to get the free info on racking.

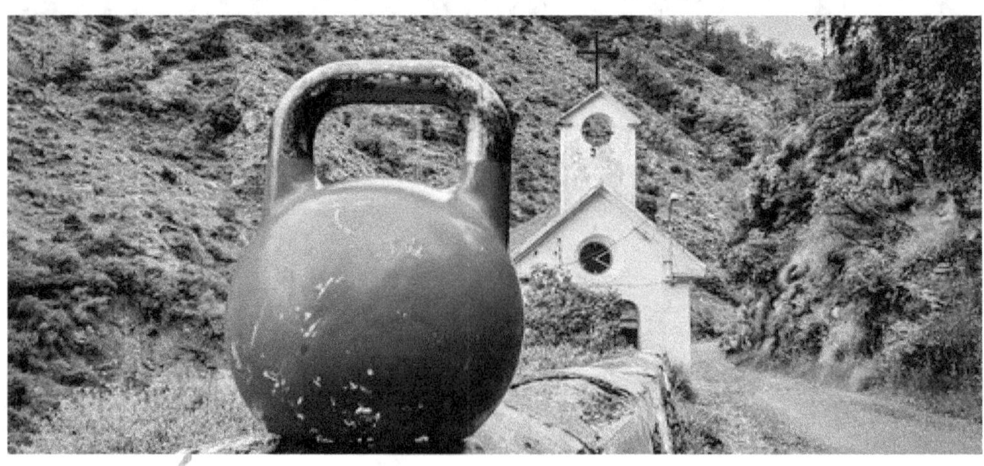

Racking Safety Grip

With this grip the thumb is over the index finger which are placed over the horn, and the remaining fingers are tucked behind the handle, this grip is used when working with Two kettlebells to protect the fingers from getting caught between the two kettlebell handles.

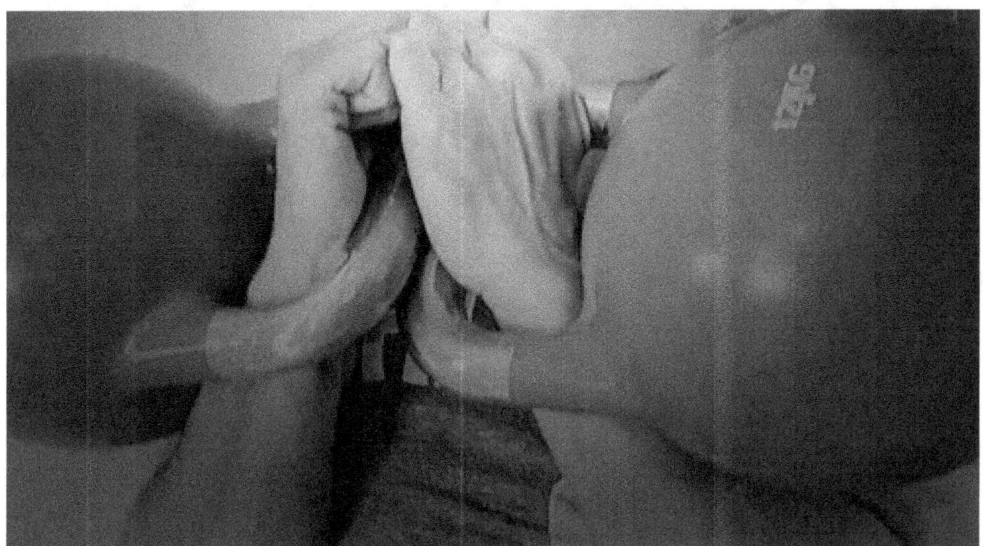

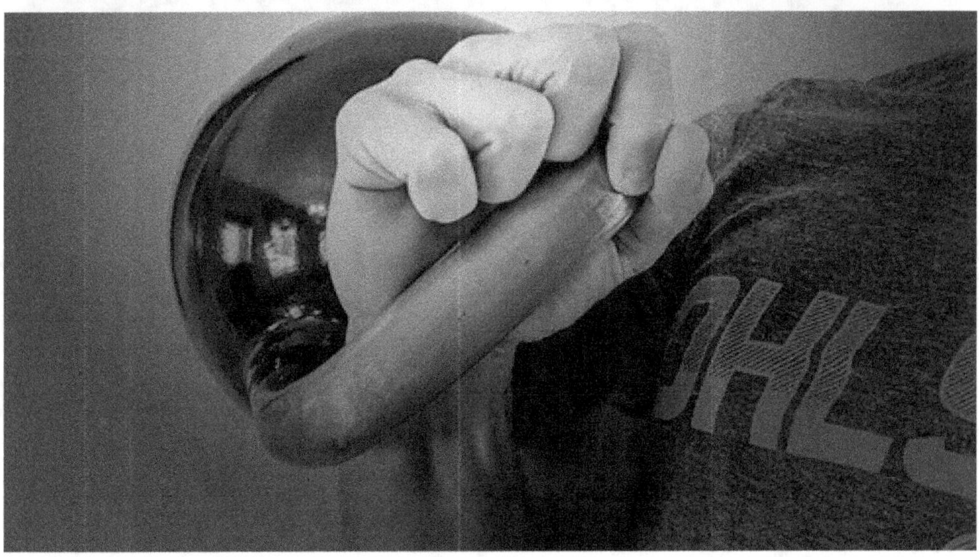

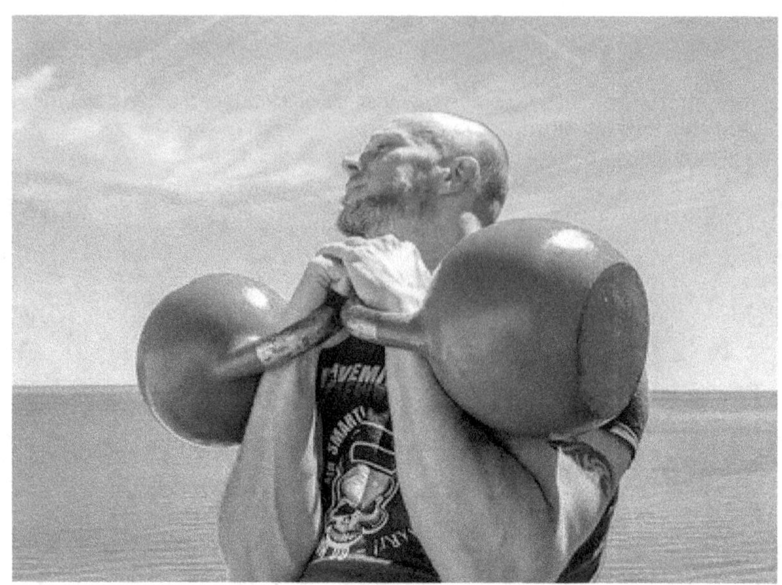

Racking safety grip

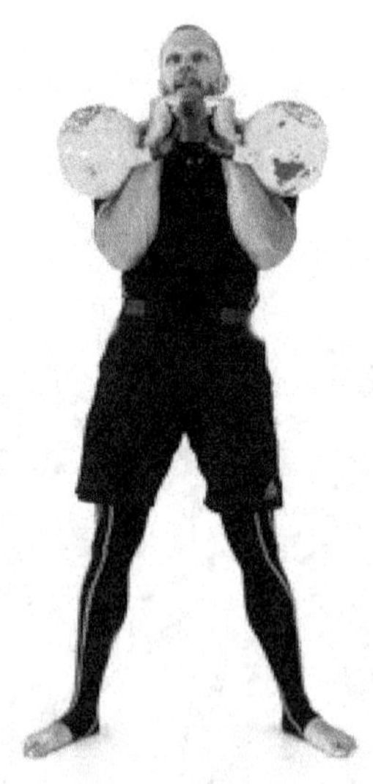

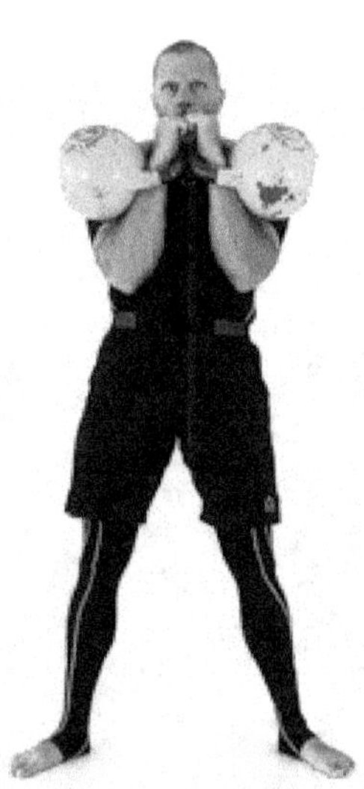

Flat Hand Grip

The hand is flat or straight with all fingers pointing up and the thumb is around the horn. Can be employed for safety with two kettlebells, racking or in overhead lock-out.

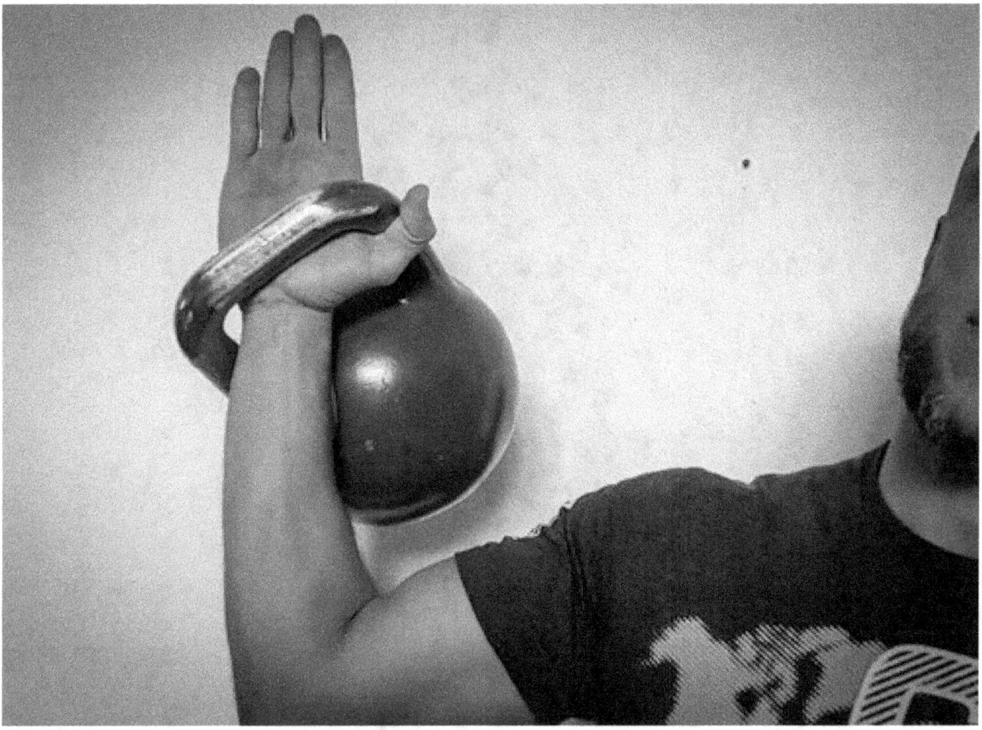

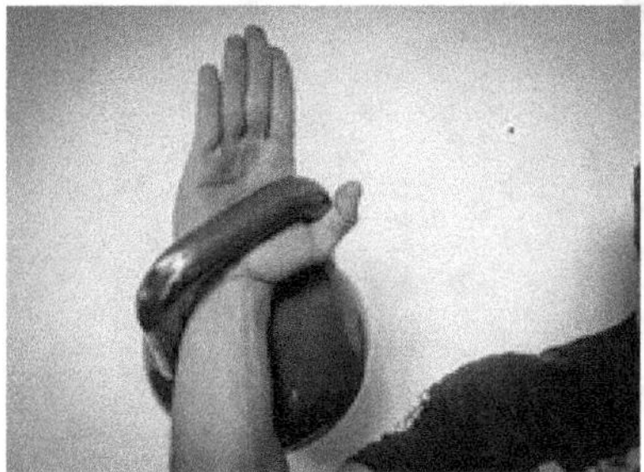

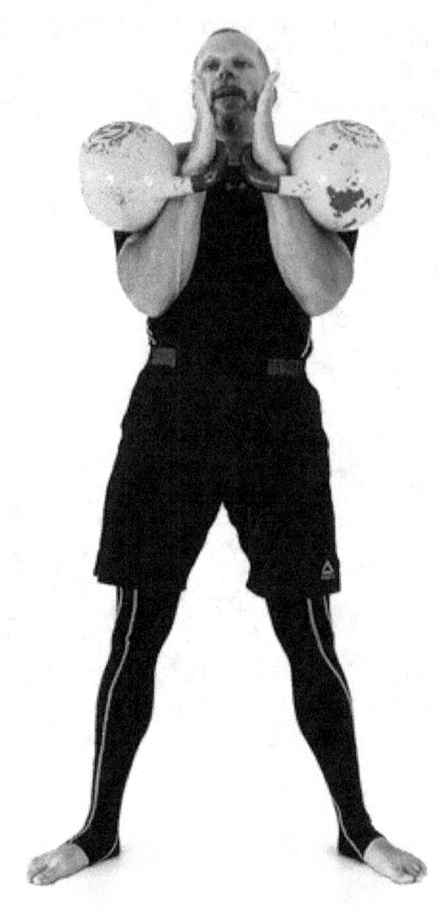

Pinch Grip

With this grip the thumb and fingers are used to pick up the kettlebell by the base of the kettlebell, this can only be performed with a smaller classic kettlebell. Used for working grip strength.

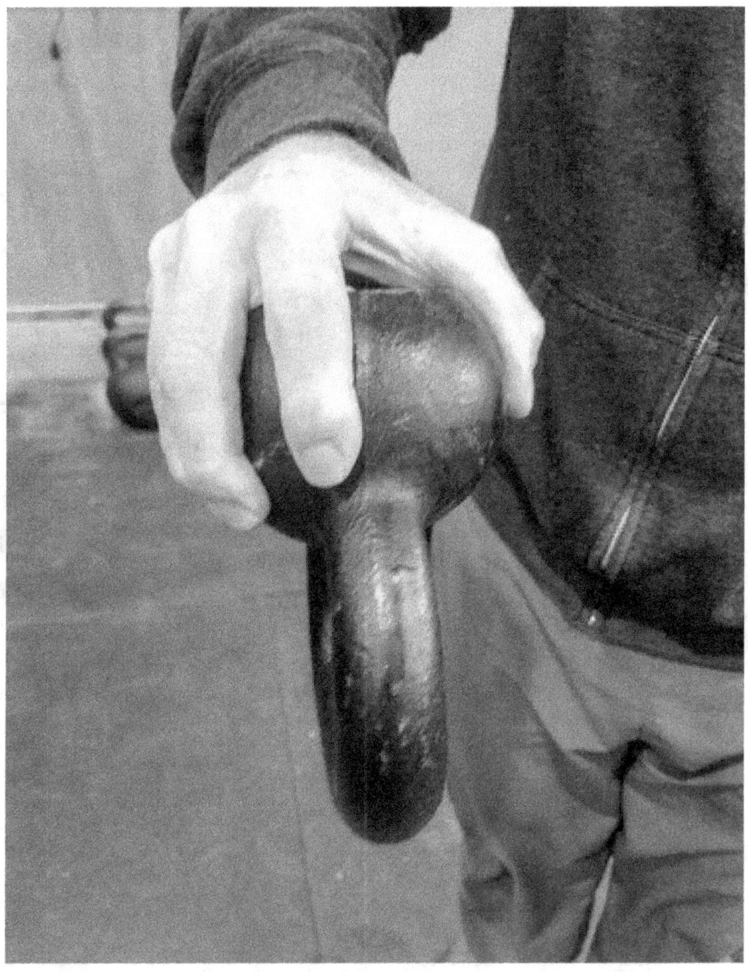

Photo provided by Robert Gagnon SFG II
www.RobGagnon.com

Farmer Grip

Grip: middle of the handle.

Handle: one hand, four fingers and thumb locking the index finger down, or both the index and middle finger

Ideal for: farmer walks, suitcase dead lifts

With this grip, the hand is placed in the middle of the handle, and used when carrying a heavy Kettlebell beside the body with farmer walks or dead lifts. It should be noted that although the farmer walk grip is usually with a firm grip —contrary to most other grips— you can perform farmer walks with a hook grip as well to challenge the fingers more.

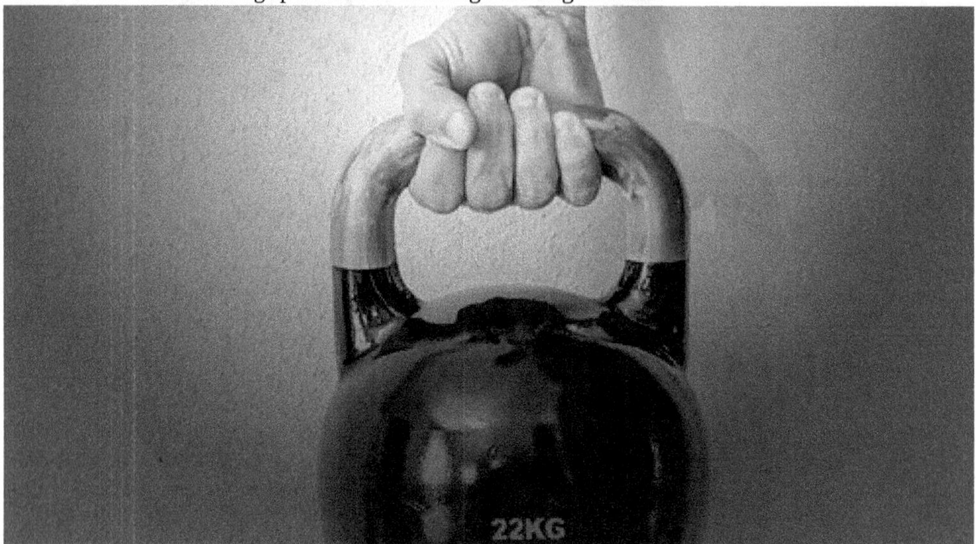

Farmer walks in action: https://www.youtube.com/watch?v=jqs8NGg50C0

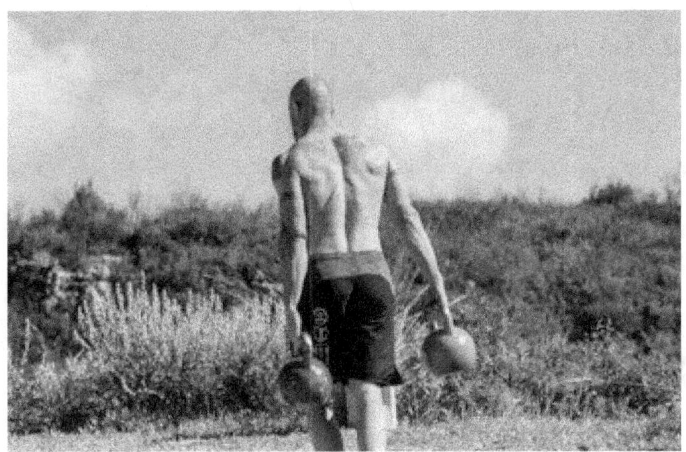

Farmer walks near Barranco Blanco on the Costa del Sol

Tip of the Fingers Grip AKA Gorilla Grip

Grip: tip of the fingers.

Handle: the handle lays in the tips of the fingers which are shaped like when manicuring the finger nails.

Ideal for: farmer walks, suitcase dead lifts, dead lifts

This grip, is an awesome grip to work on grip strength, I personally started using this to improve my grip strength for BJJ (martial art) and baptised it the Gorilla Grip. The handle should nearly be falling of the fingers that's how little grip should be used. The thumb is not used, just the four finger tips.

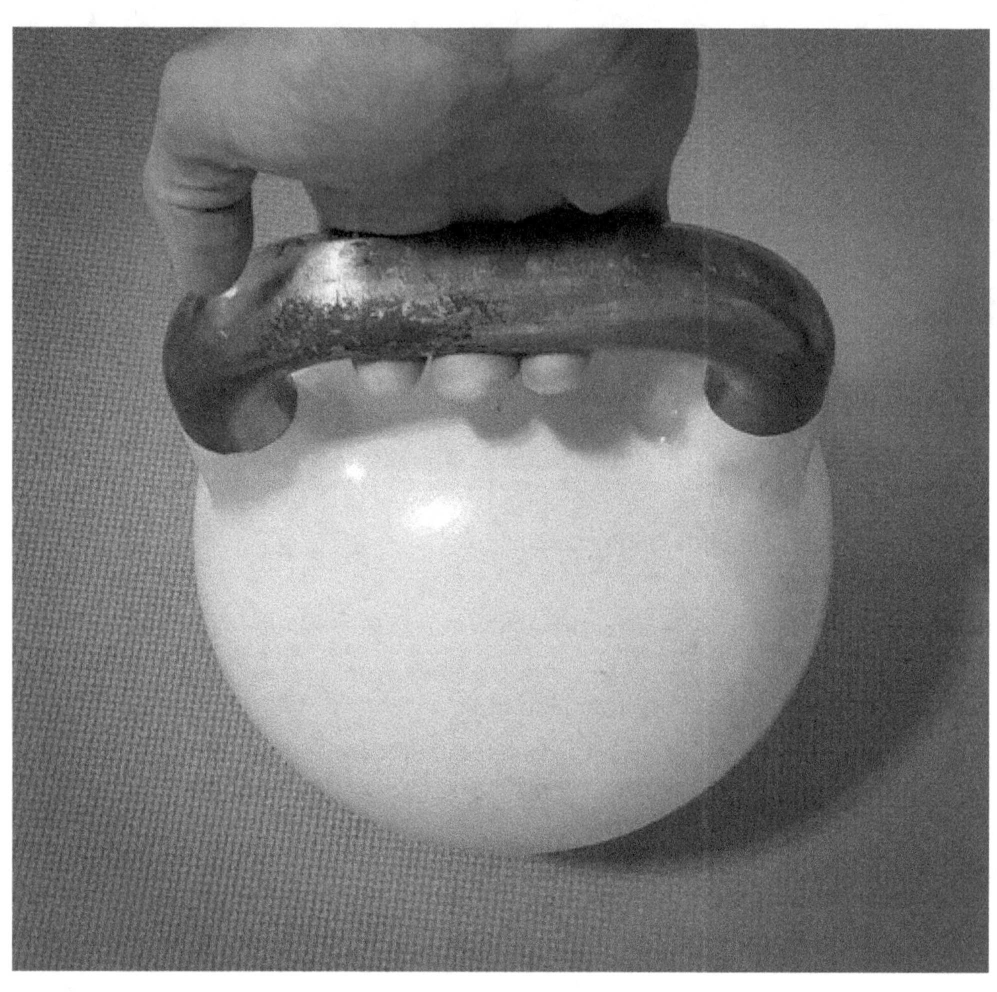

Bottoms Up Grip

Handle: one hand, four fingers and thumb crushing the handle

Ideal for: bottoms up press, bottoms up squat

This grip is performed with a strong and firm grip on the handle while the Kettlebell is upside down, and used for bottoms up press or bottoms up Turkish get-up. The bottoms-up grip is great to work on grip strength and stability.

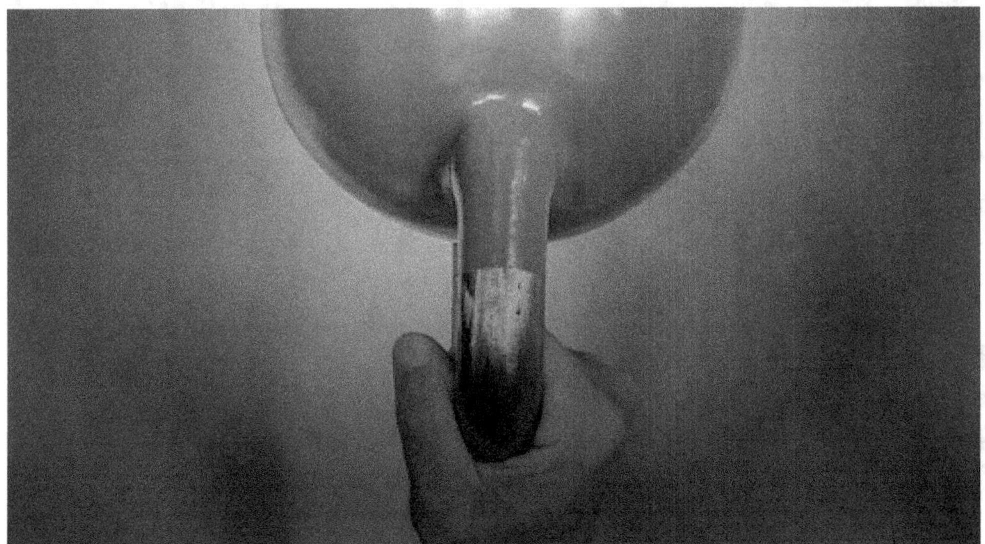

Horn Grip

Handle: two hands, four fingers and thumb locking the index finger down on the horns

Ideal for: curls, lunge and twist, halo's

This grip is performed with both hands holding the horns, and is used for doing halo's and bicep curls.

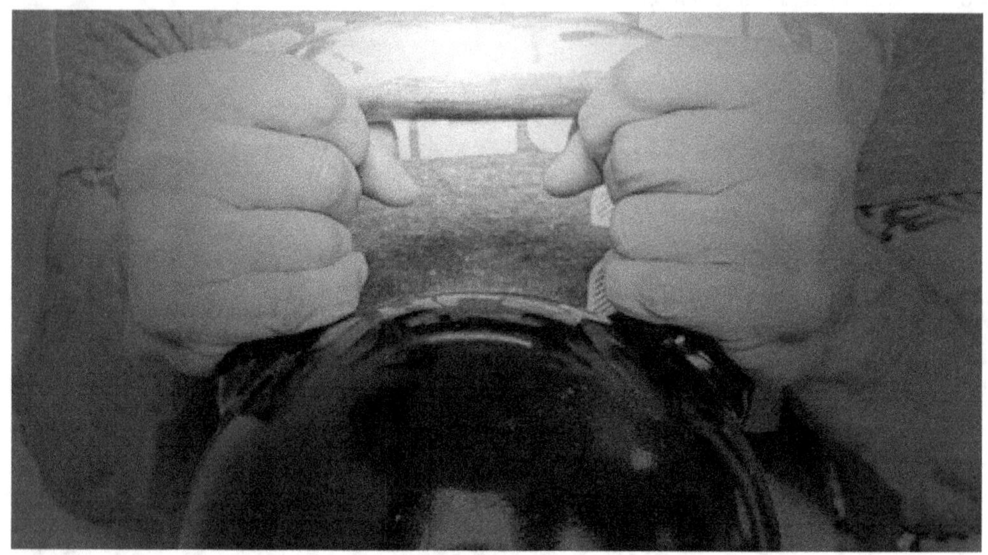

Russian twist in action: https://www.youtube.com/watch?v=_KbZno3KZdY

Horn Grip Upside Down

Handle: two hands, four fingers and thumb locking the index finger down on the horns

Ideal for: Russian twists, pull overs, halo's

This grip is performed with the hands holding the horns while the kettlebell is upside down, and can be used for pull-overs and Russian twists.

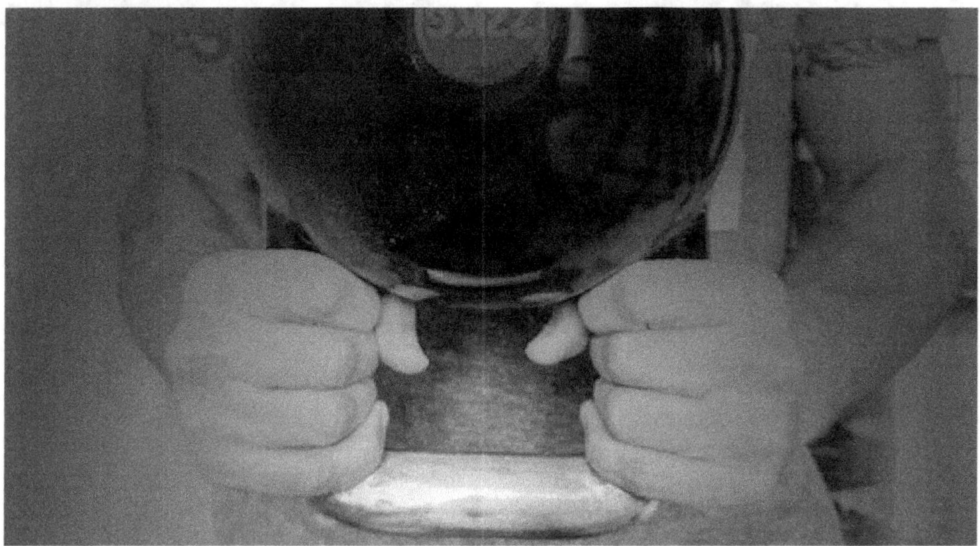

This is also a great grip to work on wrist strength with lateral wrist movement, you can do this in the air with a light bell or have the handle resting on the ground with a heavier bell. When resting the handle on the ground and base is up, the objective is to slowly move the bell forward to where it almost touches the ground, slowly and controlled bringing it back towards you as far as possible.

If you do this drill in the air it also works your biceps as you need to hold the forearms just above horizontal in a static position while moving the wrists. Of course, this will also require you to activate your lats, chest, back and abdominal muscles to provide a solid base where to perform this drill from.

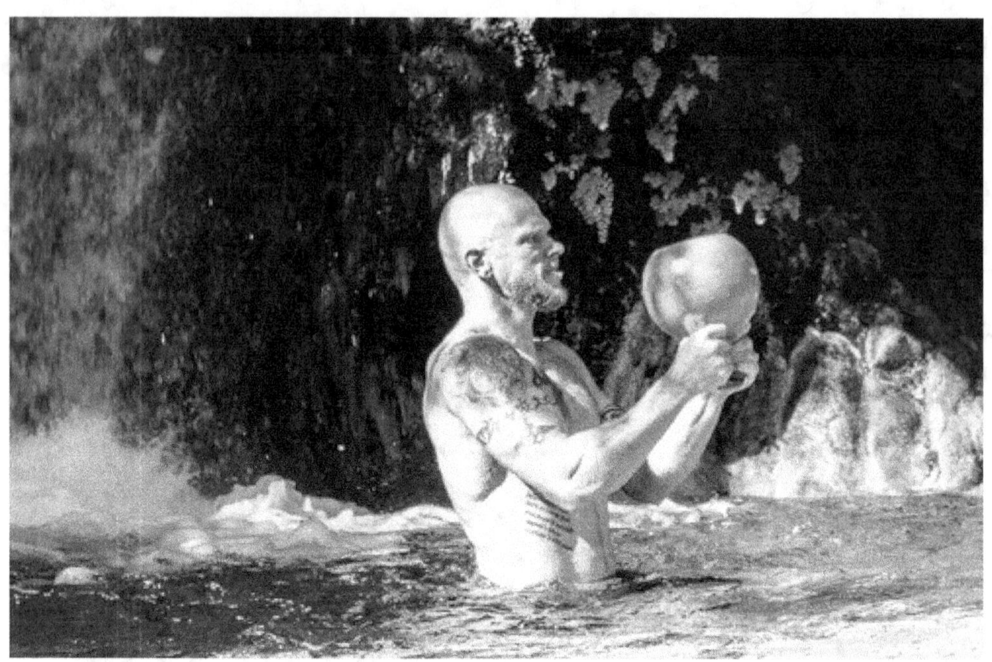

Corner Grip

Handle: one hand, four fingers and thumb loose or locking the index finger down

Ideal for: around the body, figure eight

This grip is performed with the hand holding the handle in the corner, i.e. where the handle and horn intersects, used for around the body and figure eight's. A corner grip is mostly employed for passing the kettlebell to the other hand, whether you're juggling or switching arms.

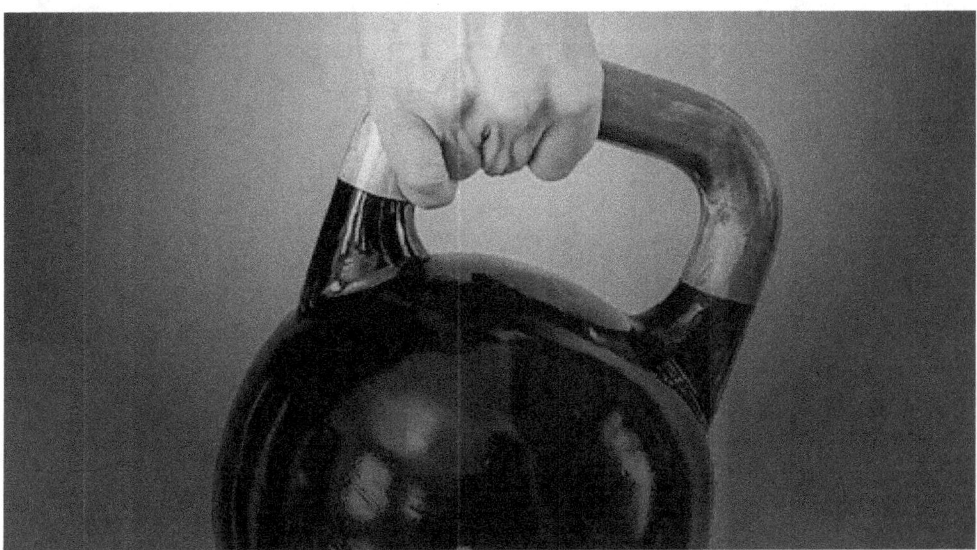

Corner grips with or without a finger lock like demonstrated in the following photo can also be used for single arm swings and snatches. Having your hand positioned there means it's already where it needs to end up in overhead position.

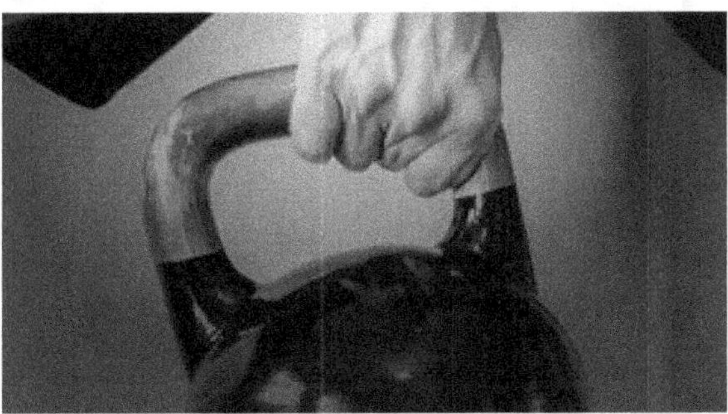

Open Hand Horn Grip

Handle: two hands, all fingers slightly squeezing the bell and the thumbs folded around the bottom of the horns

Ideal for: laying down chest presses, front squats, skull crushers

With this grip both hands are used, palms are open and slightly squeezing the bell which is resting within the palms, the thumbs are folded around the bottom of the horns. This grip is used for front squats and skull crushers.

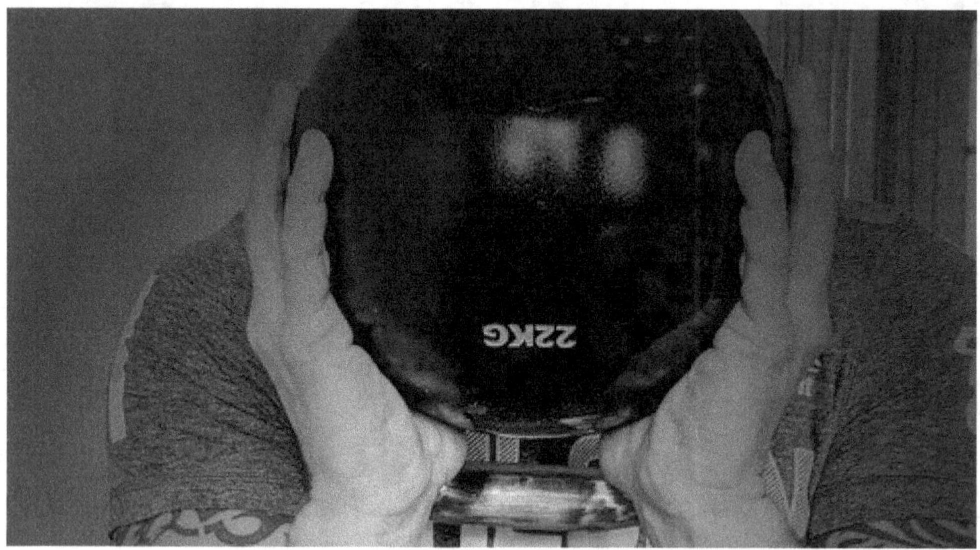

Loose Grip

Handle: one hand, four fingers and thumb loosely around the handle

Ideal for: any press variation, any overhead work, racking

This grip is performed by keeping your fingers loose rather than tightly closed and squeezing, it's used for the overhead position like presses and snatches.

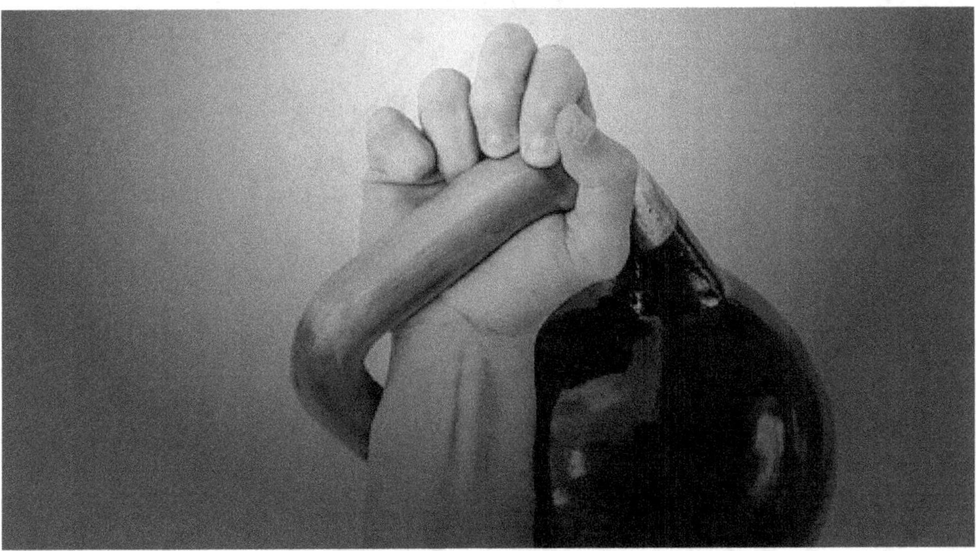

A great analogy to get the idea across for CrossFitters is thinking about a false grip.

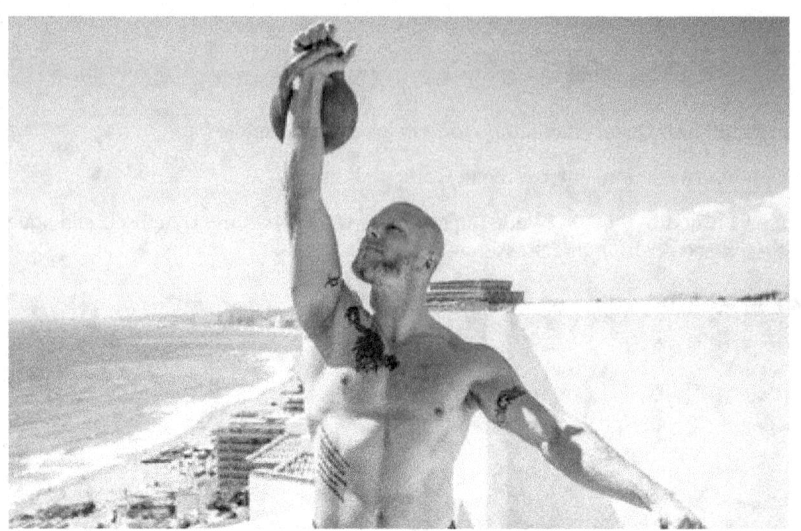

Interlocking Grip

Handle: two hands, all fingers interlocking and thumb through the corners

Ideal for: racking rest, anything performed with a rack, front squats

This grip is performed by interlocking the fingers of both hands, elbows tight into the side of the body, and is used for front squats or racked lunges.

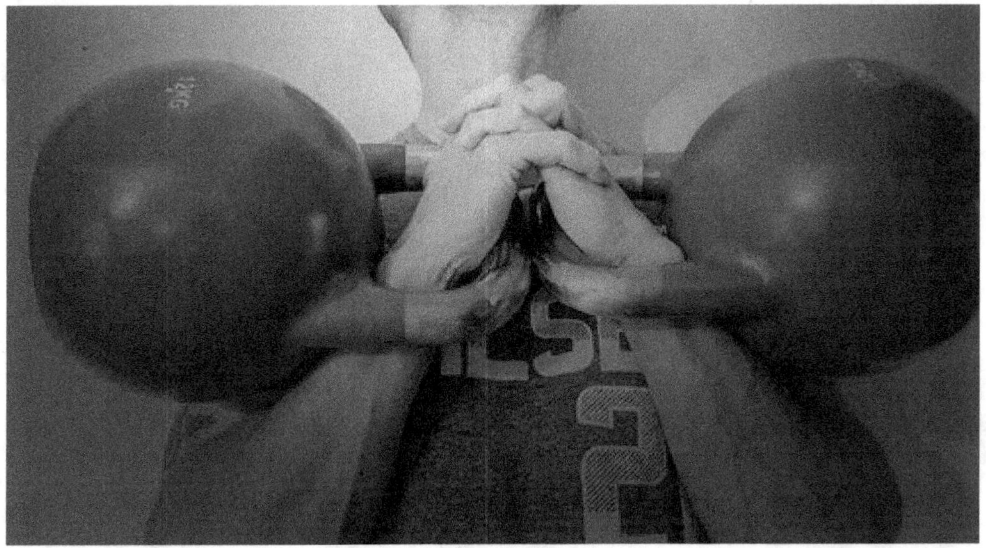

Stacking Grip

Handle: two hands, several fingers holding on to the handle of the stacked kettlebell

Ideal for: racking rest, anything going rack to overhead

This grip is performed by placing the handles on top of each other and several fingers holding on to the second handle while the top hand is over the bottom hand, used for resting or anything going overhead like the press, push press or jerk.

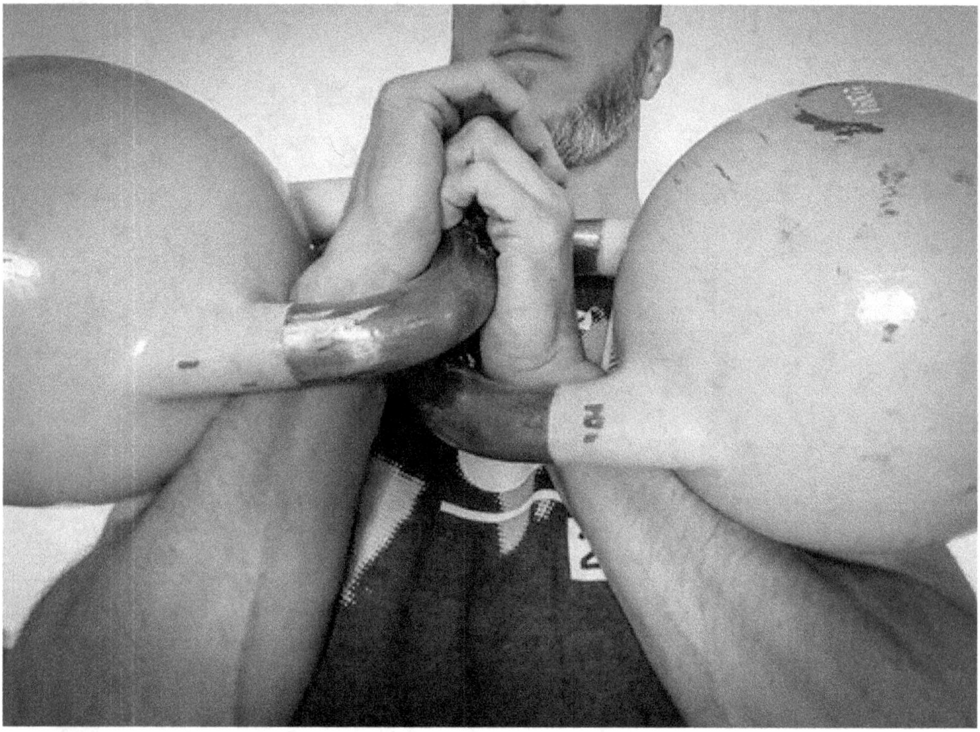

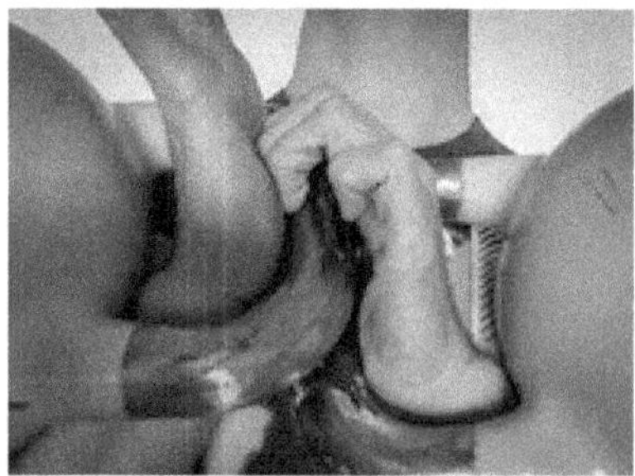

Open Palm Grip

Handle: handle is resting against the underside of the forearm

Ideal for: increasing difficulty of presses

This grip is performed with the bell resting in the open palm and handle against the underside of the forearm. Great for working on wrist strength.

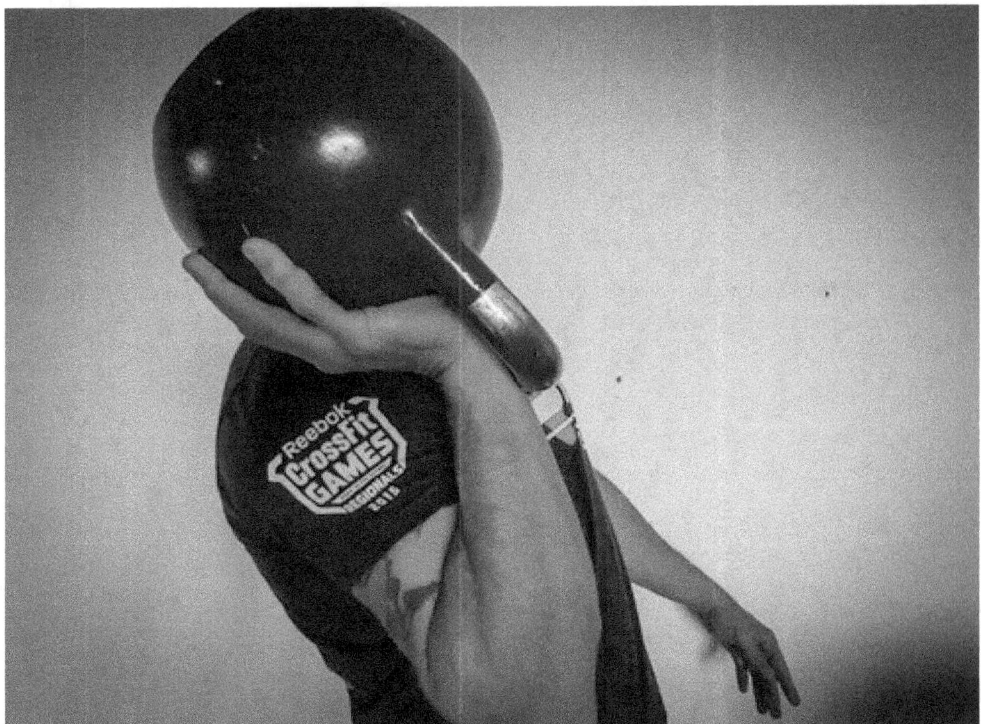

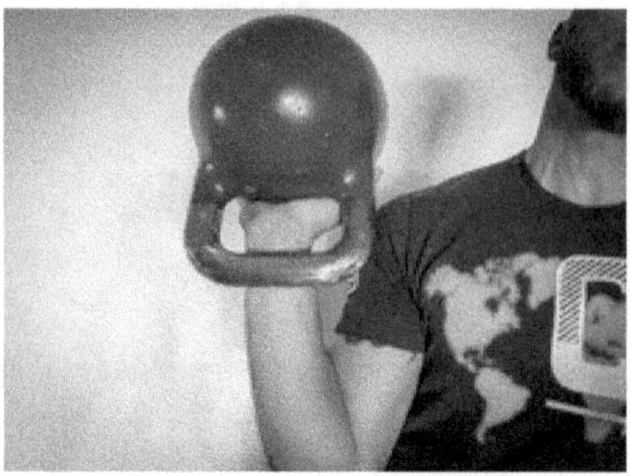

Open palm snatch in action: go.cavemantraining.com/kbe-vid-136

Waiters Grip

Handle: the handle does not come into play

Ideal for: increasing difficulty of presses

This grip is performed with the base resting on the open palm. Great for working on wrist strength. This grip is named for obvious reasons, the way the kettlebell rests on the palm resembles that of a waiter carrying a tray.

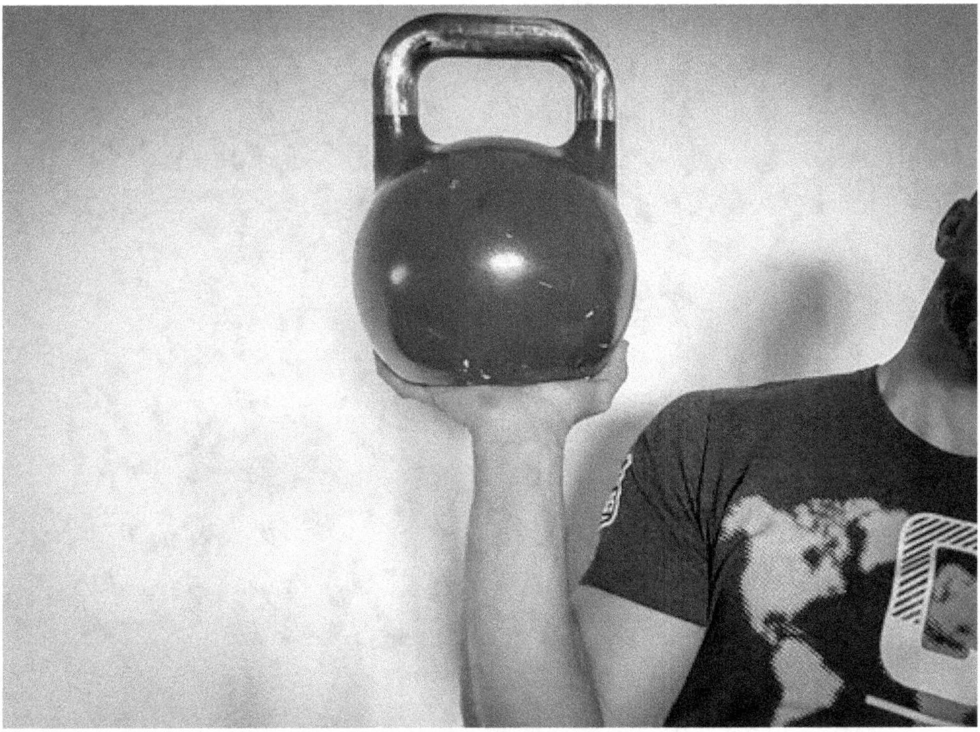

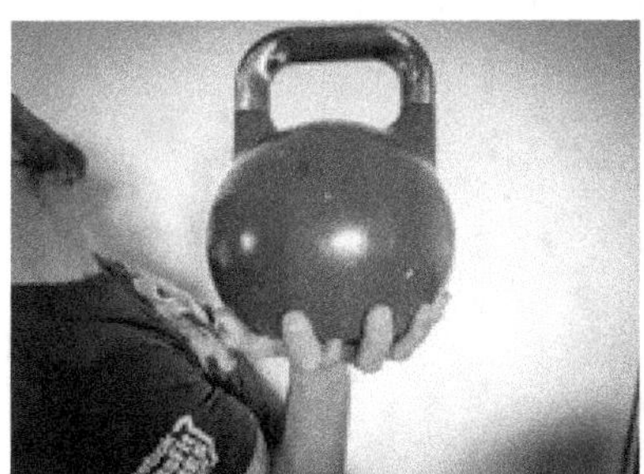 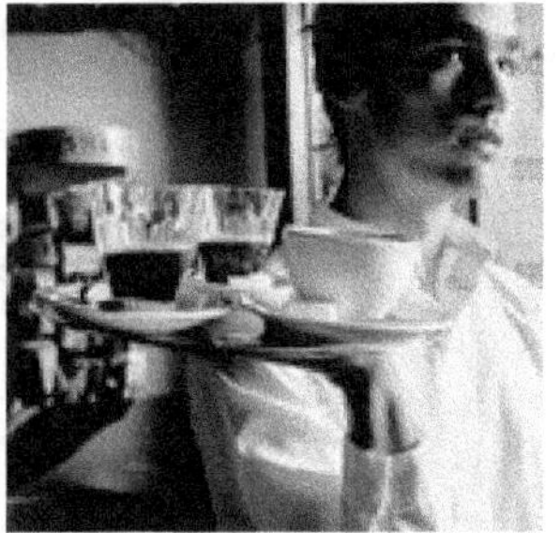

Illustrated is the waiters grip from different angle and a waiter carrying a tray

Once you get into kettlebell juggling you can swing and catch the kettlebell directly into waiters grip, from there you can perform an overhead squat. This variation requires a more explosive swing to get the kettlebell high and flip into waiters grip.

You can see the waiters grip in action here: go.cavemantraining.com/kbe-vid-137

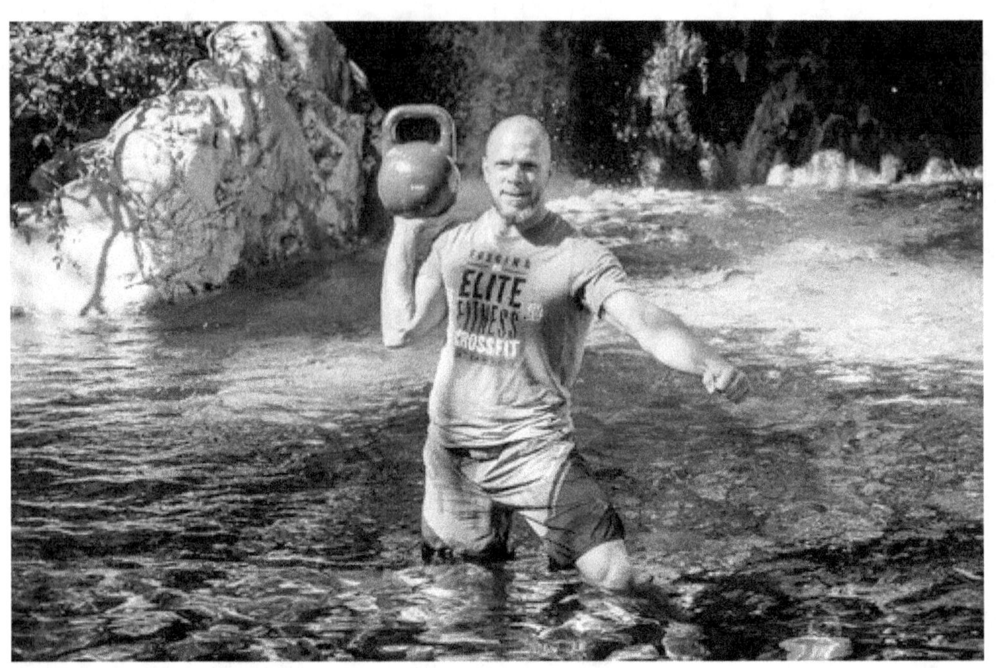

Goblet Grip

Handle: the handle does not come into play

Ideal for: front-squat

This grip is performed with the palms pressing around the bell, the handle is up or down. The grip is named for obvious reasons, the shape of the kettlebell with handle down resembles that of a goblet. With the handle facing up this grip is called the *reverse goblet grip*. The higher you go up the bell with your palms, the harder you need to squeeze, palms towards the bottom and the bell is resting more within the palms.

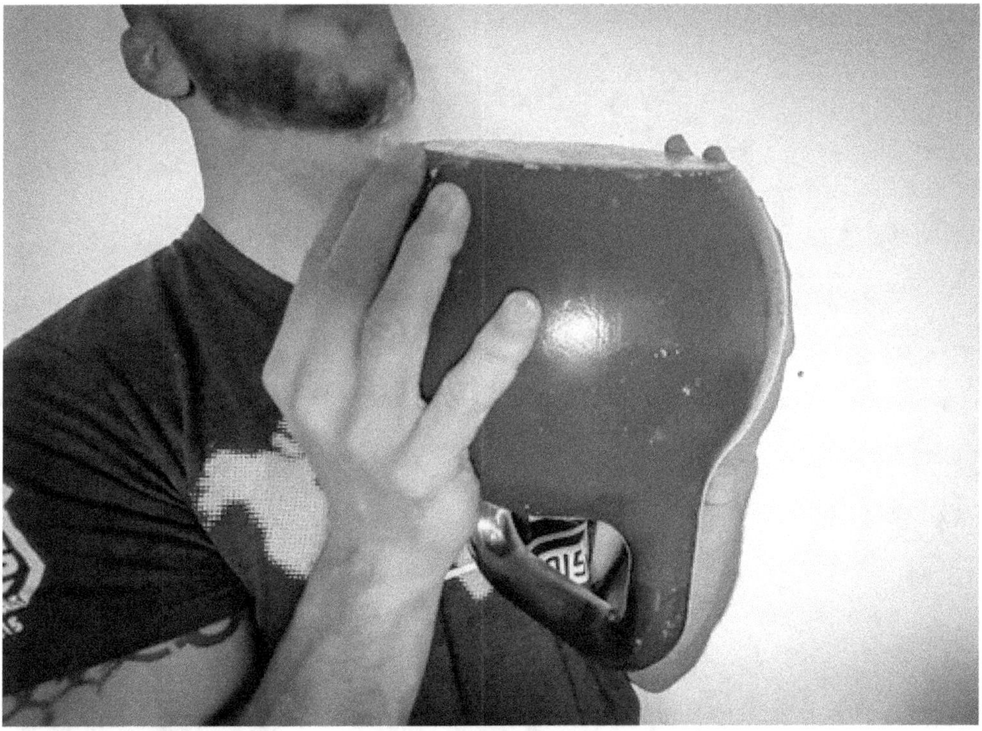

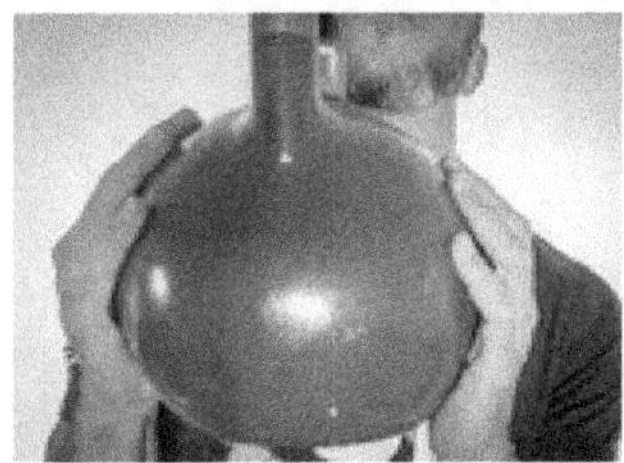

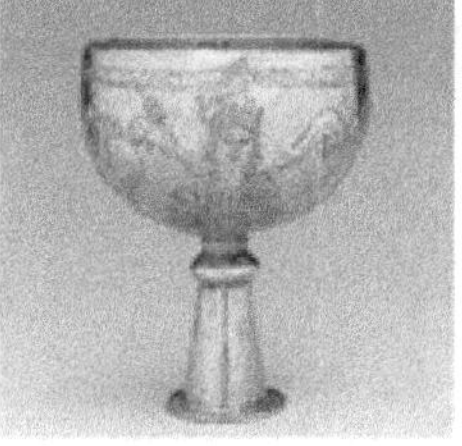

You can watch a video demonstrating the *goblet grip* in a *goblet squat.*
go.cavemantraining.com/kbe-vid-138

Crush Grip

Handle: the handle does not come into play

Ideal for: front-squat, static hold, push-up

This grip is performed with the palms crushing the bell, the handle is up or down. Similar to the goblet grip but more crushing with the palms. Great for working the pectoralis.

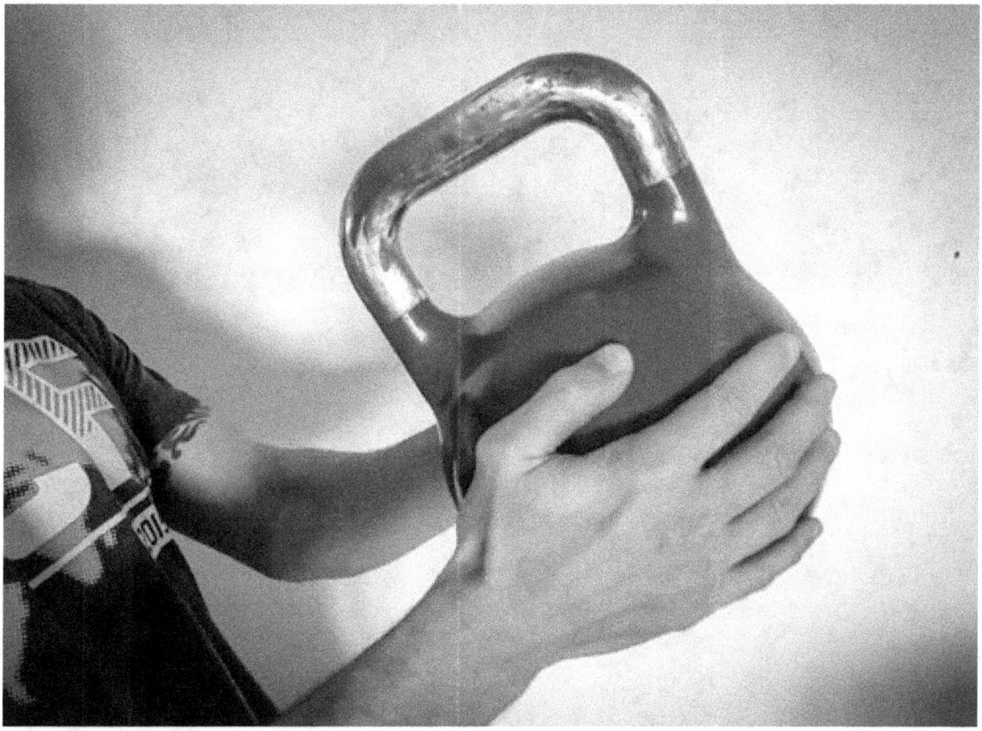

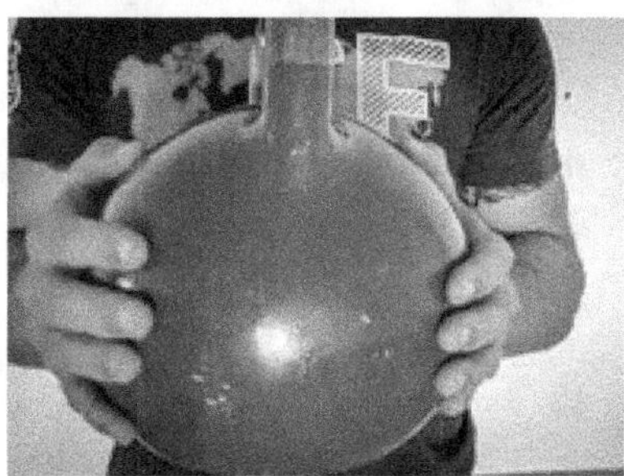

Have you tried the *kettlebell crush push-up* yet?

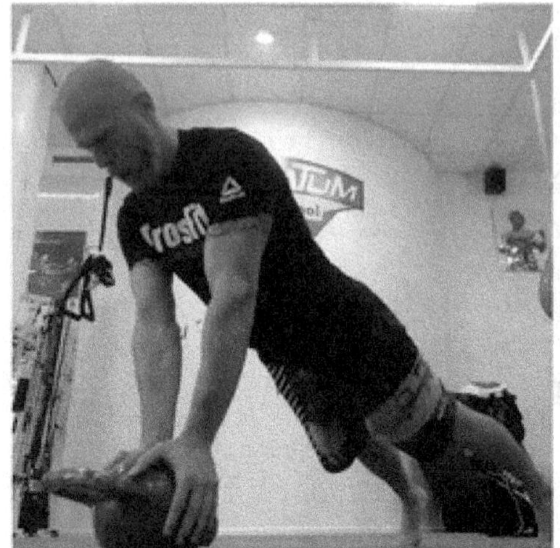
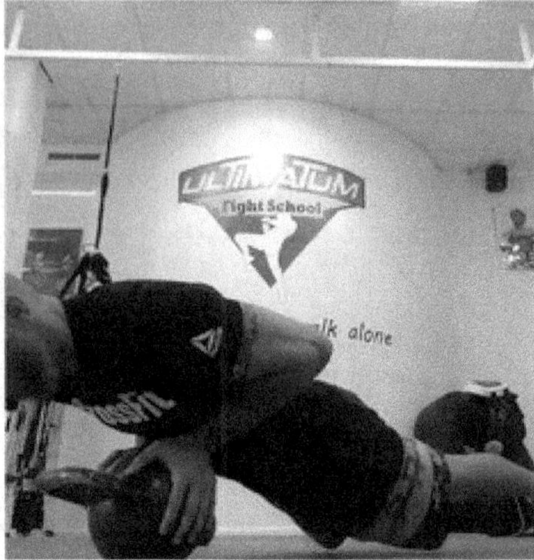

You can watch a short video here: go.cavemantraining.com/kbe-vid-139

Thumb Grip (AKA Noob Grip)

Handle: the handle is resting more on the heel of the thumb than with the loose grip.

Ideal for: press

The bell rests on the inside of the arm, complete opposite of the loose grip, the handle is resting more on the heel of the thumb. Great for shifting the weight from the outside of the arm to the inside. Full range reps from racking are not possible with this grip. Try this one with the side press starting above the shoulder and returning above the shoulder.

I like to call this the noob grip as this is the grip a lot of new people use the first ever time they lift a kettlebell without instruction.

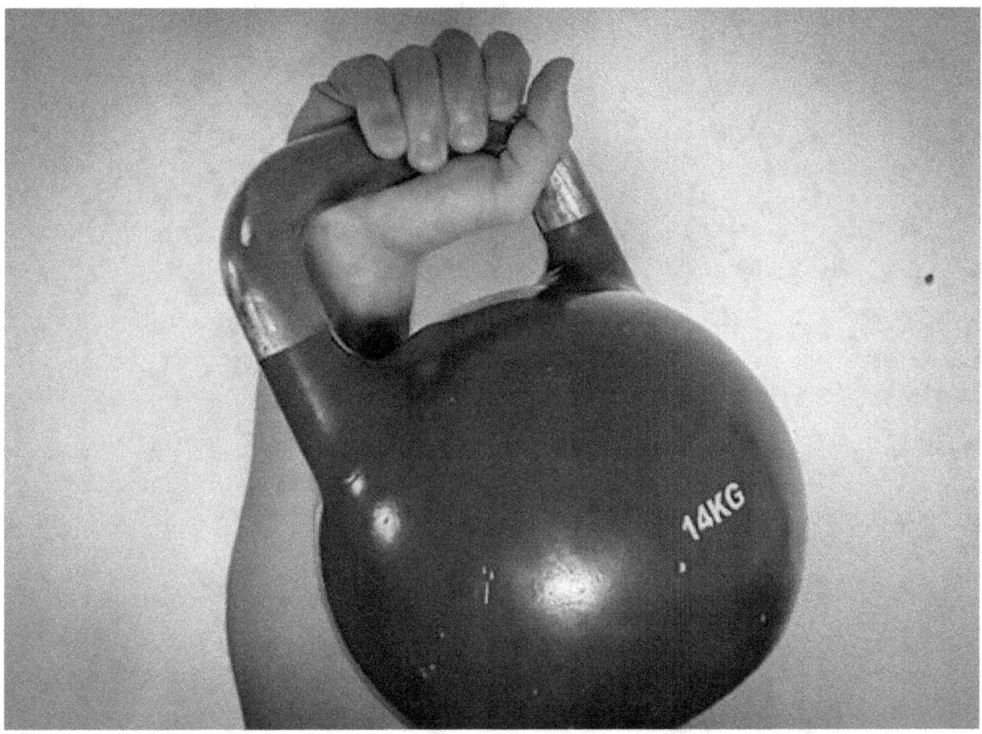

Find out why I named this the *noob grip* and why it's such a great grip to employ after you learned all other grips. www.cavemantraining.com/caveman-kettlebells/24-unconventional-kettlebell-exercises-three-broken/

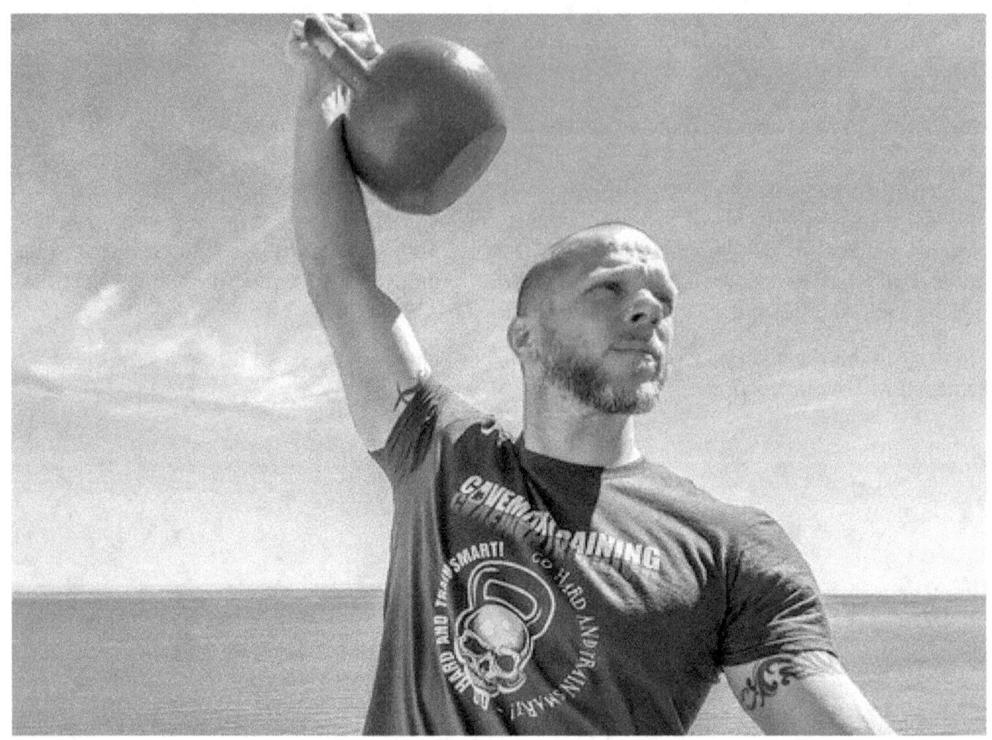

Noob grip press

More info about the *noob grip squat* can be found here www.cavemantraining.com/caveman-kettlebells/even-kettlebell-squat-bro/

Check out the combination of noob grip squat and press, try it yourself and notice the instability it provides, which is great once you've gained some strength and technique by implementing common grips. go.cavemantraining.com/kbe-vid-140

Fireman's Grip

This grip is solely used for carrying the kettlebells on or over the shoulders and is what I call the fireman's grip due to the close resemblance of the fireman's carry. With this grip your hand is holding the handle in the middle and is resting more in the fingers, the elbows are up and the kettlebell is resting on or over your shoulder. Can be performed with one or two kettlebells, one on each side.

Great for back squats, i.e. the weight is resting on the back rather than the front, can also be used for just carrying the kettlebells and walking.

Watch a demonstration of the Fireman's Squat in the following video go.cavemantraining.com/kbe-vid-141

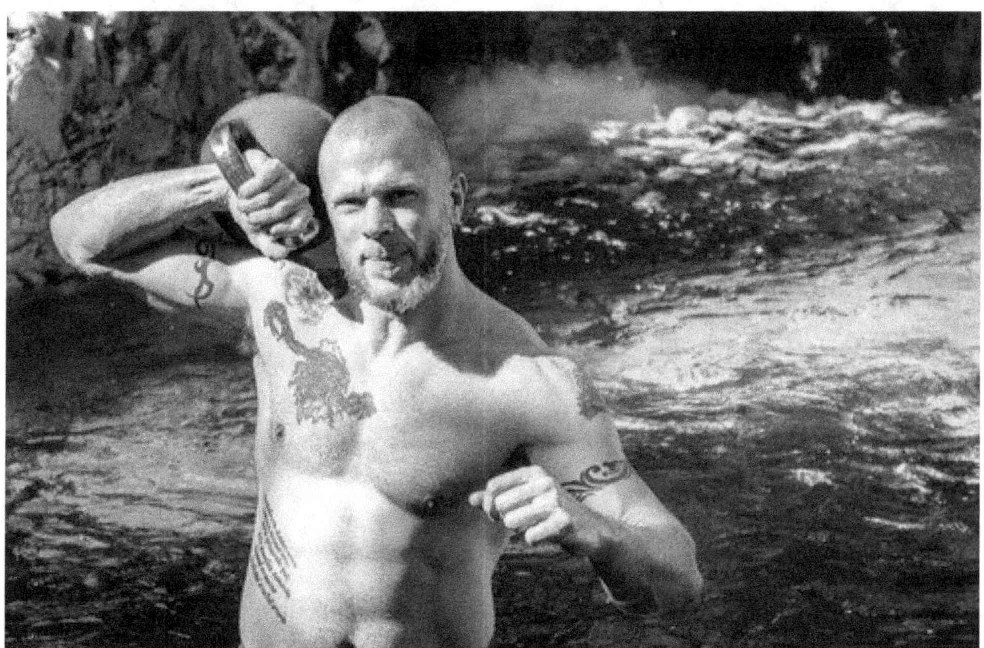

Stacked Grip

This grip is used to work with **multiple** kettlebells in one hand. It's a great grip to add more weight to your deadlifts or overhead work. The grip requires a lot more grip strength as well, as double or triple handles/weight will require more grip strength.

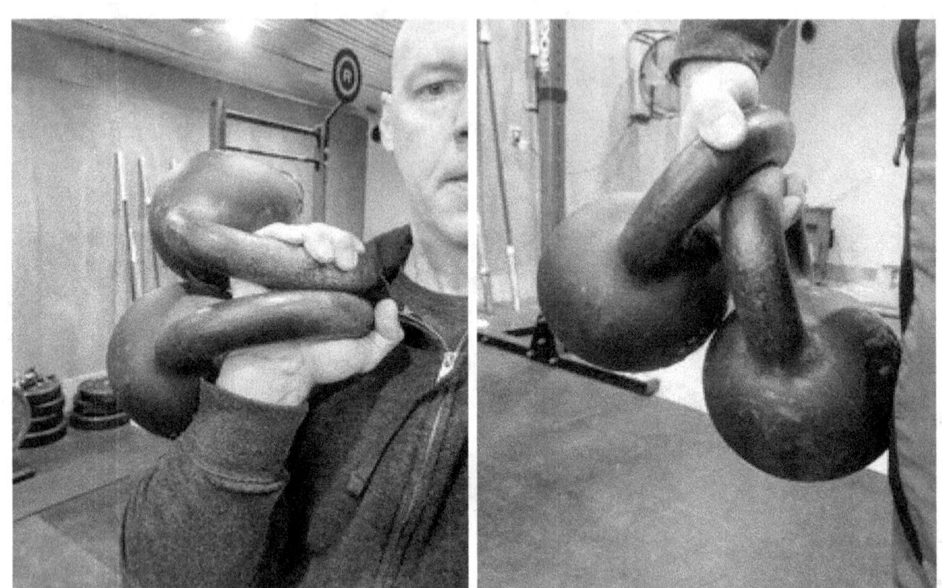

Photo provided by Robert Gagnon SFG II
www.RobGagnon.com

NOTE

If you experience forearm bruising, tenderness or pain from bell pressure, make sure you check out my detailed article on this topic, you won't find anything more detailed and intricate about this issue elsewhere. Search Google for 'Cavemantraining forearm pressure, bruising and pain'.

Other Kettlebell/Fitness Books

Other kettlebell books by Cavemantraining are:
* Kettlebell Guide For Beginners
* Kettlebell Training Fundamentals
* Kettlebell Training Fundamentals (Spanish)
* Master The Hip Hinge
* Master The Basic Kettlebell Swing
* Master The Kettlebell Clean
* Master The Kettlebell Press
* Kettlebell Workouts And Challenges 1.0
* Kettlebell Workouts And Challenges 2.0
* Kettlebell Strength Program Prometheus
* Snatch Physics
* Kettlebells For Mobility And Flexibility
* Caveman Mobility Program
* Flexibility, Mobility, And Strength Without Yoga

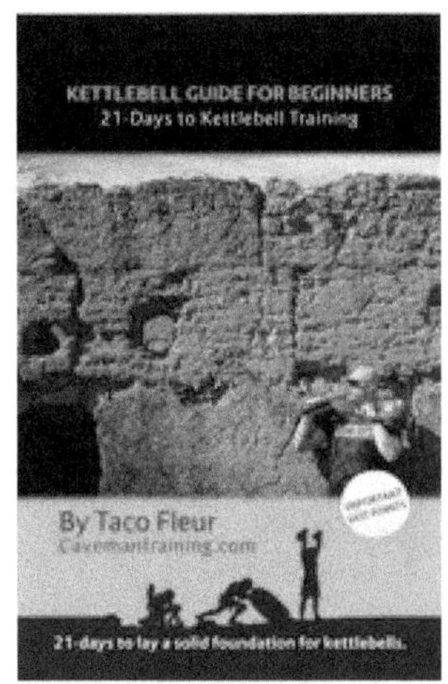

This kettlebell training book is a quick introduction to kettlebell training for beginners with dot points rather than lengthy explanations.

Buy on Amazon go.cavemantraining.com/amazon-1
Prime Video go.cavemantraining.com/amazon-2
DVD go.cavemantraining.com/amazon-3
Blu-ray go.cavemantraining.com/amazon-4
Udemy course go.cavemantraining.com/udemy-1

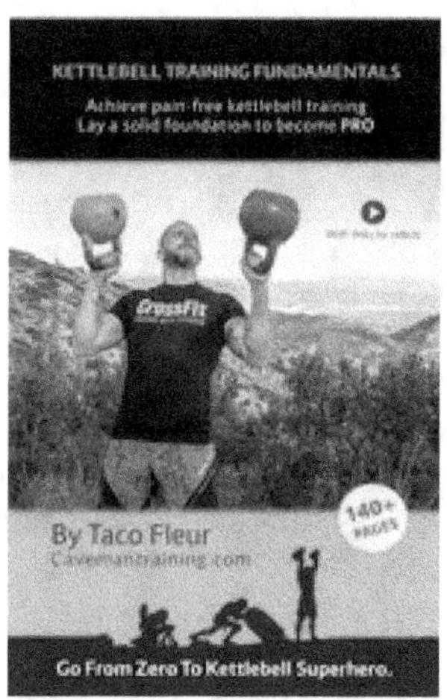

If you're looking to get into kettlebell training then there is no better book than Kettlebell Training Fundamentals, one of the best books for kettlebell training beginners to pick up and lay the proper foundations for a lifelong kettlebell journey. If you want to progress in kettlebell training then you need to master the basics, these are the basics of kettlebell training and they take you step-by-step to where you want to be, performing the fundamentals movements of kettlebell training safely and effectively. **Buy on Amazon**. go.cavemantraining.com/amazon-5
Direct download. go.cavemantraining.com/download-1

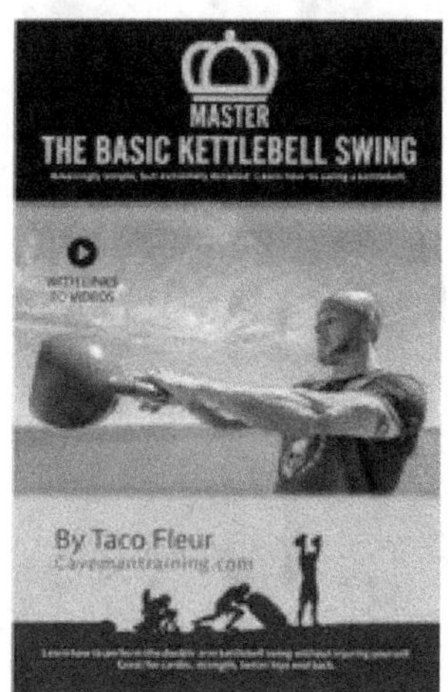

This book is your first step to becoming a serious kettlebell trainer or kettlebell enthusiast. Improve your cardiovascular endurance and potentially irradiate neck and back pain with one simple exercise. If you're a Crossfitter and want to get more efficient at snatching and the American Swing, then learn the foundation for both, the conventional kettlebell swing AKA Russian Swing. **Buy on Amazon**. go.cavemantraining.com/amazon-6
Direct download. go.cavemantraining.com/download-2

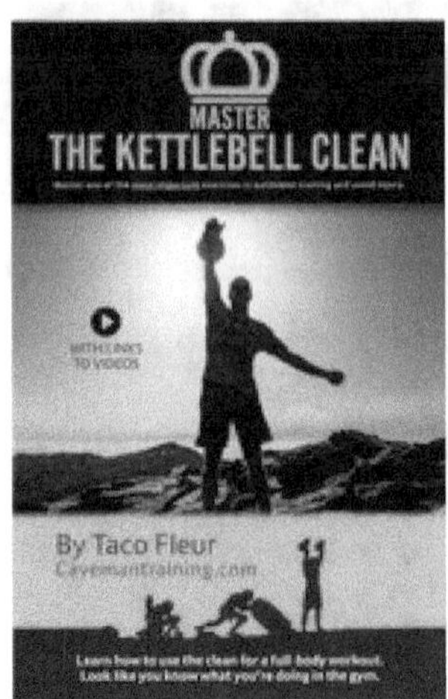

If you want to get into kettlebell training, you can't go past the clean, as simple as this exercise might sound, there is a whole lot involved, and is usually an area in which beginners get injured. I will cover most common injuries and how to avoid them.
Buy on Amazon. go.cavemantraining.com/amazon-7
Direct download. go.cavemantraining.com/download-3

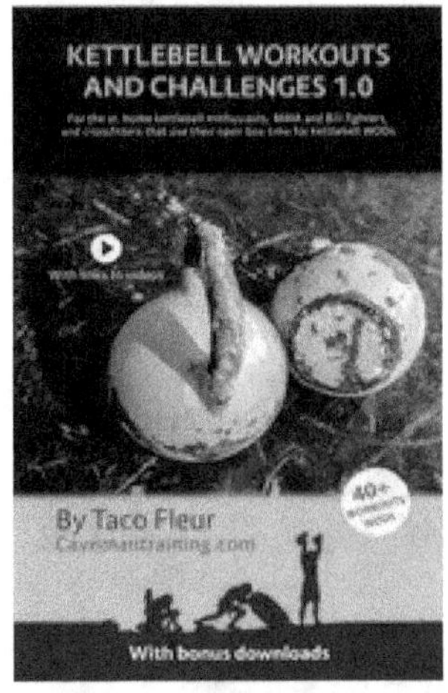

40+ serious kettlebell workouts, 4 kettlebell challenges, many are paired with very detailed videos.
Buy on Amazon. go.cavemantraining.com/amazon-8
Direct download. go.cavemantraining.com/download-4

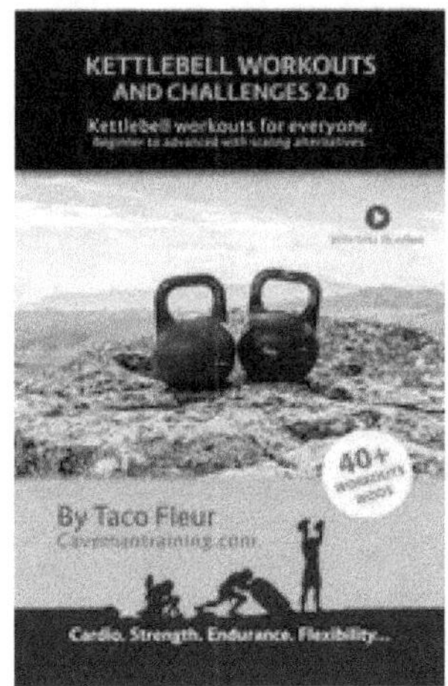

This book is targeted to at-home kettlebell enthusiasts, MMA and BJJ fighters, and crossfitters that use their open box time for kettlebell WODs. This book is even for budding trainers who want to know more about the Cavemantraining programs, and learn the basics on how to run them. 40+ serious kettlebell workouts and several kettlebell challenges, many paired with very detailed videos.
Buy on Amazon. go.cavemantraining.com/amazon-9
Direct download. go.cavemantraining.com/download-5

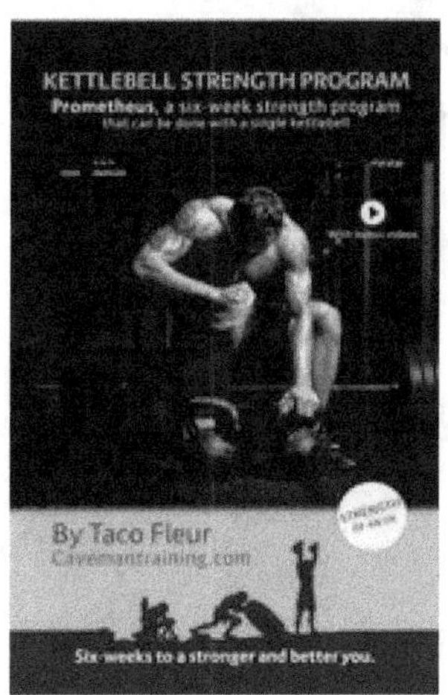

A six-week kettlebell strength program that can be completed with a single kettlebell. The program is simple and based on three super-powerful kettlebell exercises that work the full-body.
Buy on Amazon. go.cavemantraining.com/amazon-10
Direct download. go.cavemantraining.com/download-6

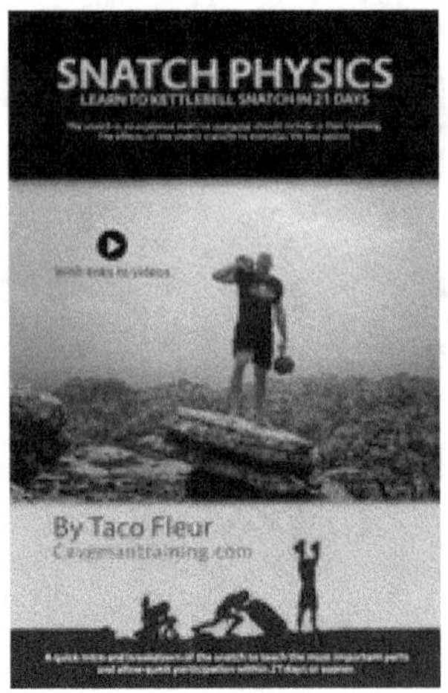

The kettlebell snatch is a full body exercise that delivers amazing effects. The snatch can be used to increase cardiovascular endurance, muscular endurance, strength, flexibility, core stability, explosive power, and much more. The snatch truly works each and every major joint in the body, ankles, knees, hips, shoulders, elbow, and wrists. For strength, you can't deny the major areas that will improve, such as, latissimus dorsi, deltoid, triceps, erector spinae, abdominals, glute, hamstrings, calves, hip flexors, quadriceps, lumbrical muscles, and many more.
Buy on Amazon. go.cavemantraining.com/amazon-11
Direct download. go.cavemantraining.com/download-7

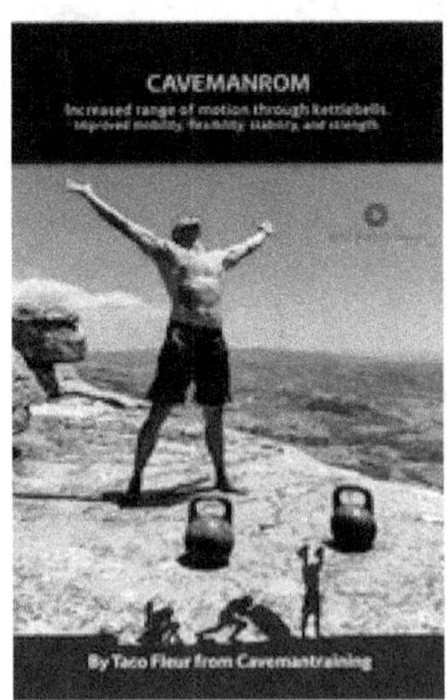

CAVEMANROM is all about loaded exercises for flexibility, stability, proprioception, strength, coordination, and everything else that increases mobility and range of motion. Injury-proof yourself. **Buy on Amazon**. go.cavemantraining.com/amazon-12

Online Kettlebell Courses

- From Zero to Kettlebell Superhero in 4 Weeks (or less)
  www.udemy.com/from-zero-to-kettlebell-superhero ~~$69.99~~
  With discount coupon: RCIL7W **$15.99**

- 21-Days to Kettlebell Training for Beginners
  www.udemy.com/kettlebell-training-for-beginners ~~$74.99~~
  With discount coupon: 5Z6P3V **$14.99**

- Kettlebell Training **PREMIUM**
  www.udemy.com/kettlebell-training ~~$149.99~~
  With discount coupon: C4DP41 **$24.99**

- Beginner Kettlebells for Females (Authored by Anna Junghans)
  www.udemy.com/kettlebells-for-females ~~$59.99~~
  With discount coupon: KRJO2E **$14.99**

- Kettlebells—A VITAL Course to Take
  www.udemy.com/kettlebell-exercise ~~$79.99~~
  With discount coupon: 98ZLUT **$14.99**

- Kettlebells for Great Looking Shoulders
  www.udemy.com/kettlebells-for-shoulder-strength ~~$39.99~~
  With discount coupon: RP8NYF **$9.99**

- Kettlebell Exercise for Cardio and Weight Loss
  www.udemy.com/kettlebell-snatch/ ~~$149.99~~
  With discount coupon: 59QI3O **$29.99**

- Kettlebell Workouts
  www.udemy.com/kettlebell-workouts ~~$74.95~~
  With discount coupon: WG7ILS **$19.99**

Online Kettlebell Certifications For Trainers

- Kettlebell Fundamentals Trainer L3.0
  www.cavemantraining.com/shop/training-course/kettlebell-fundamentals-trainer-l3-0/

- Kettlebell Snatch Trainer L3.0 + L4
  www.cavemantraining.com/shop/training-course/online-kettlebell-snatch-certification-by-cavemantraining/

- Kettlebell Clean Trainer L3.0 + L3.1
  www.cavemantraining.com/shop/training-course/kettlebell-clean-variations/

- CAVEMANROM Trainer L3.0
  www.cavemantraining.com/shop/certification/cavemanrom-trainer-online-certification/

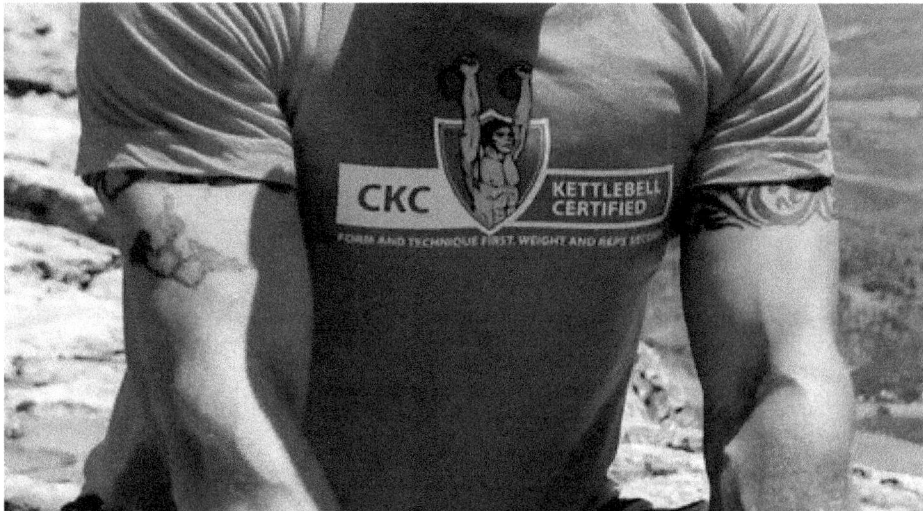

Join Us

Join *Cavemantraining* in one of the following groups/social channels:

- Kettlebell Training 11,000+ members as of 2019
  www.facebook.com/groups/KettlebellTraining/

- Kettlebell Workout 2,500 members as of 2019
  www.facebook.com/groups/kettlebell.workout/

- Kettlebell Enthusiasts 2,500 members as of 2019
  www.facebook.com/groups/kettlebell.enthusiasts/

- Kettlebell Training on Reddit
  www.reddit.com/r/kettlebell_training

- Cavemantraining on Pinterest
  pinterest.com/Cavemantraining

- Cavemantraining on YouTube
  youtube.com/Cavemantraining

- Cavemantraining on Facebook
  www.facebook.com/caveman.training/

Thank You

I would like to thank you for your purchase and I truly hope to hear or see you during your kettlebell journey, whether online or offline. If anything in this book has helped you in any way I'm always happy to hear about it. I have a passion for kettlebells but more so for bringing that knowledge across so that others can improve their lives, whether that is through gaining strength, cardio, flexibility, or confidence.

On the flip-side, I have done my best to provide you with the best instructions, but I also know that nothing is perfect, if there is something that you think can be improved I would love to hear about it. me@tacofleur.com

Huge thanks to my wife, son, and French bulldog for always being there for me, I could not have done this without any of you.

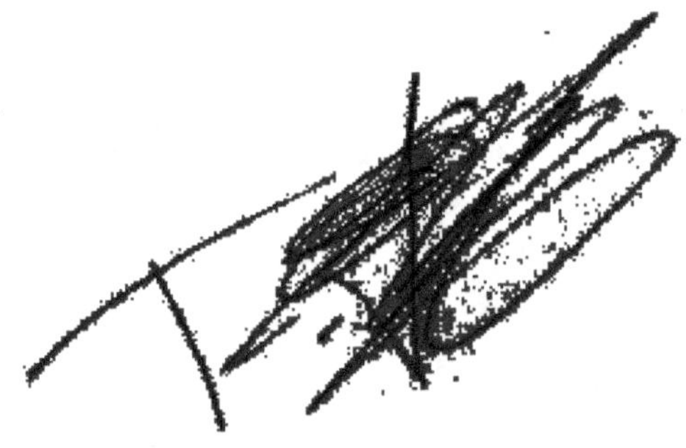